"Classified by Common Symptoms"

Meridian Exercise
for Self-Healing Book2

Ilchi Lee

"Classified by Common Symptoms"

Meridian Exercise
for Self-Healing Book2

Healing Society, Inc.
7664 W. Lake Mead Blvd. #109
Las Vegas, NV 89128

e-mail: book@healingsociety.org
Web site: www.healingplaza.com

Call 1-877-324-6425, toll-free.

Library of Congress Control Number: 2003104266
ISBN 0-9720282-8-5

Printed in South Korea

"Classified by Common Symptoms"

Meridian Exercise
for Self-Healing   Book 2

Ilchi Lee

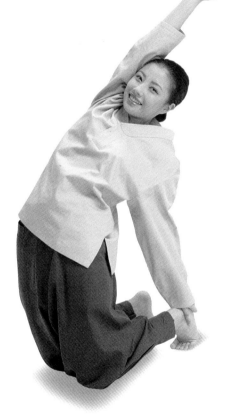

Healing Society

PREFACE

In the twenty-first century, health remains an increasingly important subject. Although cancer remedies, use of hormones to prevent aging and other medical advancements proliferate, there is no sign that incidence of illness is decreasing. Environmental pollution, food and water contamination and stress are taking an increasing toll on our bodies.

It is high time for us to re-evaluate existing medical practices. Modern medicine focuses on treatment, rather than on prevention of disease. Though state of the art treatment is important, making progress in the area of preventive medicine is far more important. Beyond the limitations of pills and surgery prescribed for symptomatic treatment, we need to adopt a holistic perspective and treat the human body as a wholly integrated organism. The human body is an organism composed of interconnected organs that profoundly affect one another. When there is a problem with the stomach, instead of reaching for a scalpel, we should examine and improve functioning of the whole body in relation to the stomach.

For the past 20 years, I have been systemizing and improving Korea's traditional training method, known as Dahnhak to fit the modern lifestyle. Research, clinical testing and practical experience confirm the effectiveness of Dahnhak in the prevention of disease and degeneration. Dahnhak strengthens the body and its natural healing power by strengthening the fundamental life force. Dahnhak Meridian exercise, is basic Dahnhak training and is a comprehensive health regimen that expands to enrich the spiritual body as well as bringing health to body and mind.

Look through the table of contents and identify your particular symptoms. Then find the specific corresponding exercises that you can perform to relieve your symptoms. The exercises in this book not only eliminate painful symptoms, but also enhance overall health to aid in prevention of disease. You may individualize your exercise program according to your particular needs. If you are experiencing specific health issues, it is advisable to consult with a health care professional before proceeding with the training.

It is most important to experience Dahnhak with your body. The methods presented here will not help you unless you experience them physically. It is through continuous practice that you will experience the benefits of Dahnhak!

Ilchi Lee

CONTENTS

BOOK 2

CONTENTS

BOOK 1

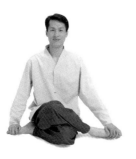

MY BODY IS NOT ME, BUT MINE

MY MIND IS NOT ME, BUT MINE

CHAPTER 4

MERIDIAN EXERCISES FOR
SPECIFIC SYMPTOMS

1. HEART AND CIRCULATORY SYSTEM

1) **HEART DISEASE**

✿

Adherents of Eastern Medicine propose that when there is an imbalance of Ki energy circulation of the heart, you can experience a sense of sadness. When there is depletion, excess, and/or a blockage of Ki energy in the heart, it can be adversely affected. A balance of Ki energy in your heart promotes a sense of joy and ebullience. When a person has heart disease, pain can be experienced in the chest and underarm area. Also, a person with this condition can exhibit irritable, rigid, and compulsive types of behavior. Emotions become unstable and can result in a constriction of the arterial flow, along with high blood pressure and heart palpitations. It is helpful to allow yourself to take a short nap during the day and relax and calm your mind effortlessly.

The Dahnhak Meridian exercises can help to improve the condition of the heart muscle and regulate improved blood and Ki energy circulation. If you have been diagnosed with heart disease, it is necessary to perform breathing in the opposite fashion to that which is normally described in the execution of the Meridian exercises. For example it is recommended that you exhale as you begin the motion and inhale to return to the original posture.

PULLING KNEE TOWARD THE CHEST (Book 1, p. 89)

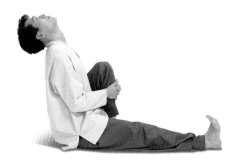

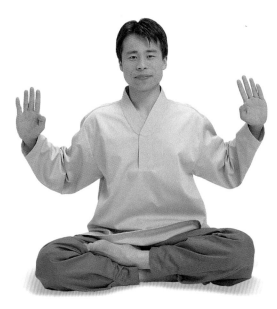

❷ Inhale. Open your hands and extend your arms as far as is comfortable keeping them at chest level. Focus on expanding your chest.

1. EXPANDING THE CHEST

Benefits Promotes deep and full breathing and enhances heart and lung capacity. Regarding STEPs 2 and 4: If you sit and hold these positions for ten minutes or more, this can help realignment of the spine and bones. Keep your spine straightened and focus on your heart. Ki and blood circulation will be strengthened, as will your heart.

TIPS If you experience palpitations or difficulty in breathing, perform the movements and just breathe naturally and comfortably.

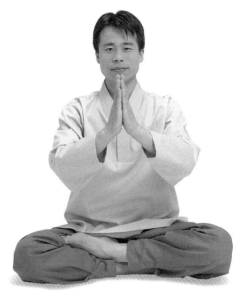

① Sit in a half-lotus postion. Place both hands in the prayer position in front of your chest.

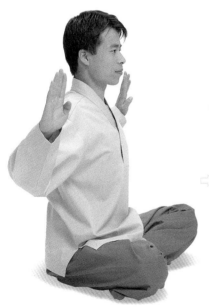

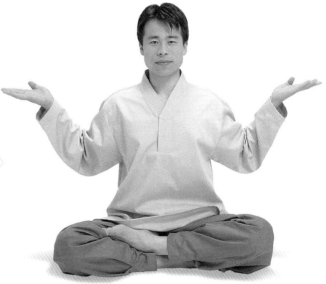

③ Keep your spine lengthened while holding your breath. Gently pull your shoulder blades towards each other and hold for ten seconds.

④ Exhale and bring your hands together in the prayer position, as in STEP 1. Inhale and slowly pull your arms apart again as far as you comfortably can with your elbows bent, and your wrists flexed. Face your palms towards the sky with your shoulders and hands parallel. Remember to keep your spine lengthened and your neck and shoulders relaxed. Focus on your heart.

2. HALF-LOTUS FORWARD BEND

Benefits Relieves tightness in chest and promotes deep and full breathing capacity.

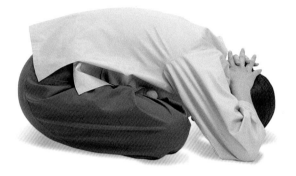

① Sit in a half-lotus postion. Lock your fingers behind your neck. Inhale. Bend your upper body forward and touch the floor with your forehead and elbows.

② Hold this position for as long as you comfortably can. Exhale and expand your chest as you return to the original posture.

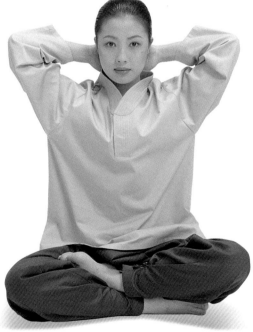

3. SITTING SIDE BEND

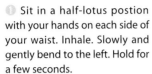 Sit in a half-lotus postion with your hands on each side of your waist. Inhale. Slowly and gently bend to the left. Hold for a few seconds.

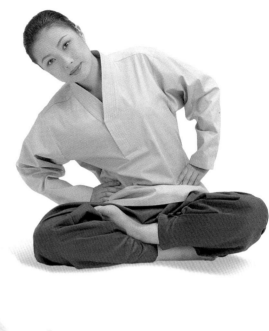

② Exhale. Inhale and bend to the right side. Hold for a few seconds. Exhale to STEP 1 original posture.

③ Repeat STEP 1 and 2 five times

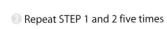

4. ARM TWIST

Benefits When you have heart difficulty you can feel stiff in the arms and shoulders. This exercise helps to release this stiffness and activates the Pericardium Meridian(see page 192, #9) and the Heart Meridian(see page 190, #5).

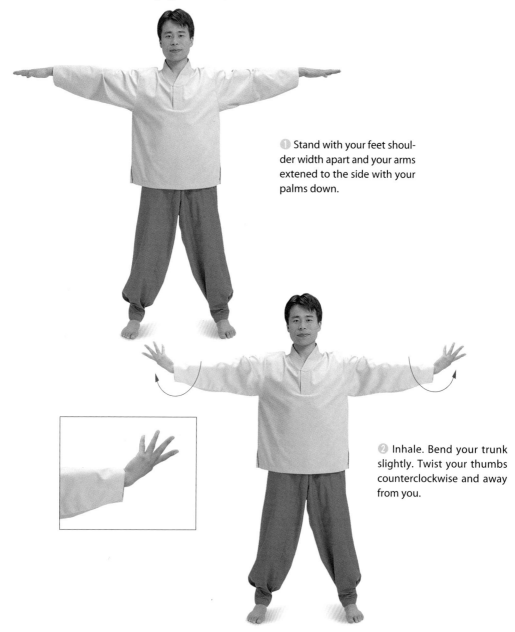

① Stand with your feet shoulder width apart and your arms extened to the side with your palms down.

② Inhale. Bend your trunk slightly. Twist your thumbs counterclockwise and away from you.

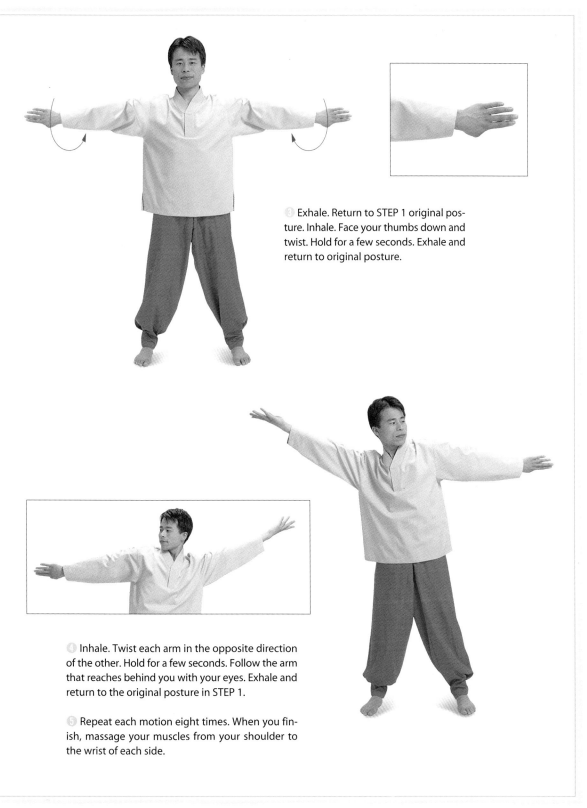

❸ Exhale. Return to STEP 1 original posture. Inhale. Face your thumbs down and twist. Hold for a few seconds. Exhale and return to original posture.

❹ Inhale. Twist each arm in the opposite direction of the other. Hold for a few seconds. Follow the arm that reaches behind you with your eyes. Exhale and return to the original posture in STEP 1.

❺ Repeat each motion eight times. When you finish, massage your muscles from your shoulder to the wrist of each side.

5. PRESSING THE YONG-CHUN ACUPRESSURE POINT

① Sit with your knees bent as shown in the picture. Make fists with both of your hands. Press the Yong-chun acupressure point with the middle joint of the third finger.

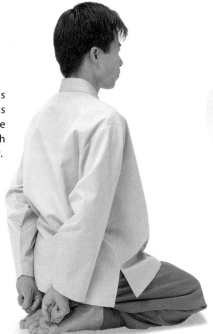

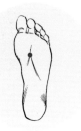

Yong-chun

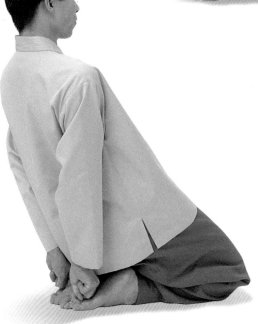

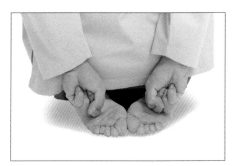

② Inhale. Gently lift your hips with your weight on your hands. Press the Yong-chun acupressure point for about seven seconds. Exhale. Repeat five times.

6. ARCHER EXERCISE

TIPS Keep your upper torso facing towards the center. Move only your head and follow movement with your eyes. Relax the neck and shoulders as you perform this exercise.

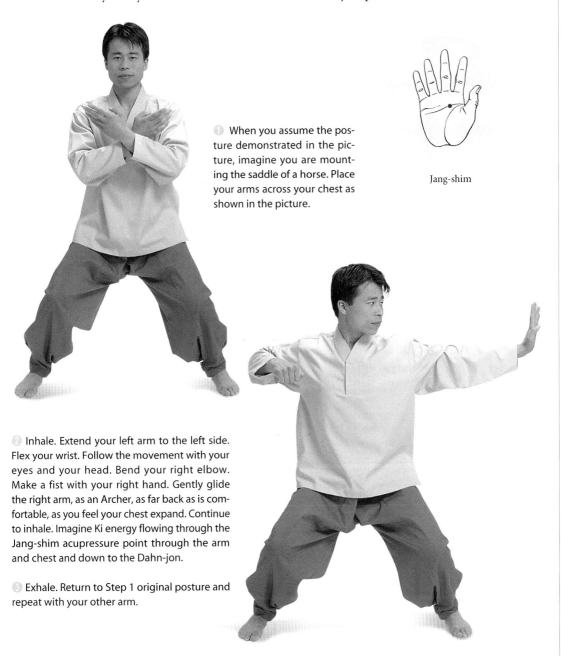

① When you assume the posture demonstrated in the picture, imagine you are mounting the saddle of a horse. Place your arms across your chest as shown in the picture.

Jang-shim

② Inhale. Extend your left arm to the left side. Flex your wrist. Follow the movement with your eyes and your head. Bend your right elbow. Make a fist with your right hand. Gently glide the right arm, as an Archer, as far back as is comfortable, as you feel your chest expand. Continue to inhale. Imagine Ki energy flowing through the Jang-shim acupressure point through the arm and chest and down to the Dahn-jon.

③ Exhale. Return to Step 1 original posture and repeat with your other arm.

7. WHOLE BODY RELAXATION

Benefits This exercise promotes relaxation of the body and mind and enhances blood circulation. Alpha brain wave function is accessed, assisting in self-healing for hypertension, insomnia and other autonomic nervous system disorders.

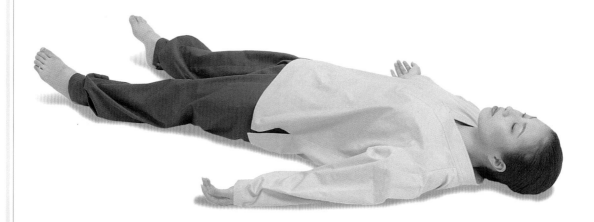

❶ Lie on your back. Place your feet shoulder width apart and your arms at a 45-degree angle, palms facing up. Close your eyes.

❷ With your mind's eye, scan your face, neck, shoulders, arms, hands, fingers, chest, Dahn-jon, back, hips, legs, feet, and toes and note where you experience tension.

❸ Imagine the bright light of the sun, melting the iced streams of winter, as you begin to see the waters now flow with the guiding light of the sun. Focus your mind upon releasing any tension you may experience in your body.

❹ Imagine now that your body is warmer and warmer and your head cooler than the rest of your body. Breathe naturally and comfortably throughout this exercise. As you become more and more relaxed, your breathing will become slower and deeper.

8. BREATHING FOR THE HEART

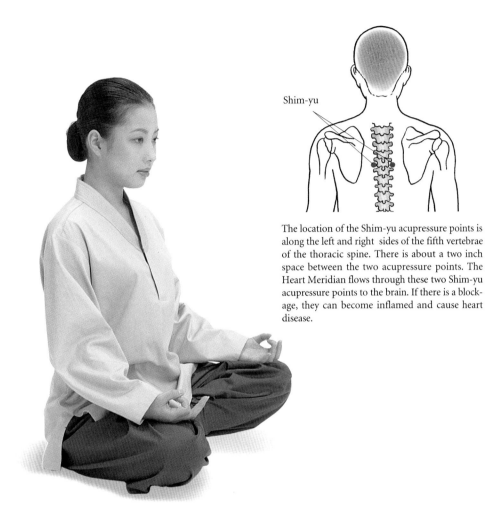

Shim-yu

The location of the Shim-yu acupressure points is along the left and right sides of the fifth vertebrae of the thoracic spine. There is about a two inch space between the two acupressure points. The Heart Meridian flows through these two Shim-yu acupressure points to the brain. If there is a blockage, they can become inflamed and cause heart disease.

To perform this exercise, sit in a half-lotus postion, with your thumbs and index fingertips touching, as shown in the picture. Focus on the Shim-yu acupressure points and the heart. Imagine the Ki energy flow connecting the heart and the Shim-yu points, as you breathe slowly and gently. Continue breathing for about fifteen to twenty minutes. As you breathe, you can experience your chest accumulating Ki energy and your heart becoming stronger and stronger.

9. HOLDING UP THE HEAVEN

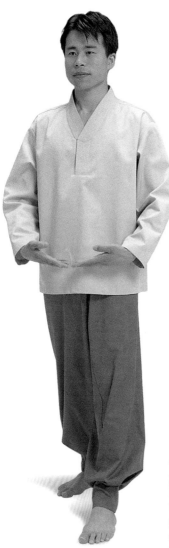

① Stand. Place your left foot straight in front of you with your right foot at a 45-degree angle. Place your hands at the vicinity of the Dahn-jon, with your palms facing up and your fingertips facing one another.

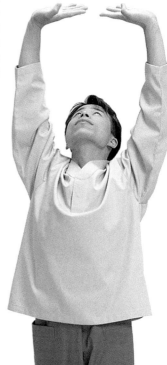

② Inhale. Gently lift your arms, with your palms facing up. Rotate your hands at chin level with your thumbs turning out and keeping your palms up, as you raise them above your head. Follow this movement with your eyes and gaze at the back of your hands.

③ Exhale. Bring your hands down to the STEP 1 original posture. Switch the position of your feet and repeat the exercise.

10. SOLE CLAPPING

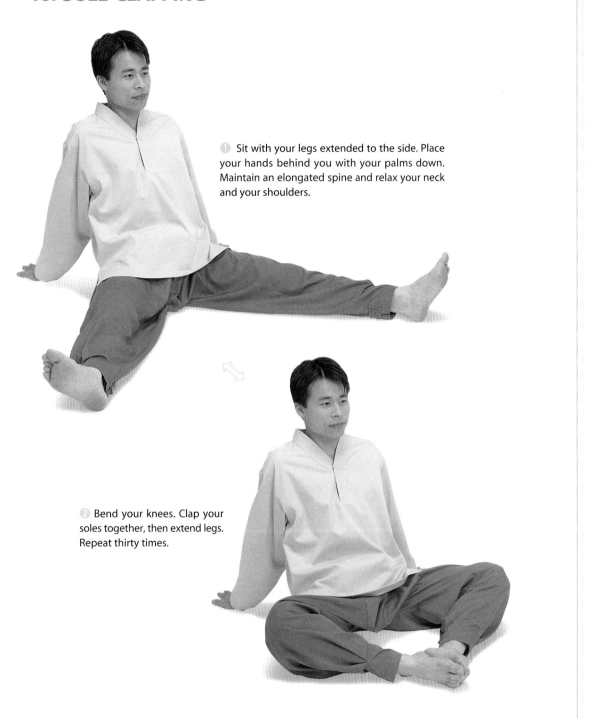

① Sit with your legs extended to the side. Place your hands behind you with your palms down. Maintain an elongated spine and relax your neck and your shoulders.

② Bend your knees. Clap your soles together, then extend legs. Repeat thirty times.

11. WAIST LIFTING WITH EXTENDED LEGS

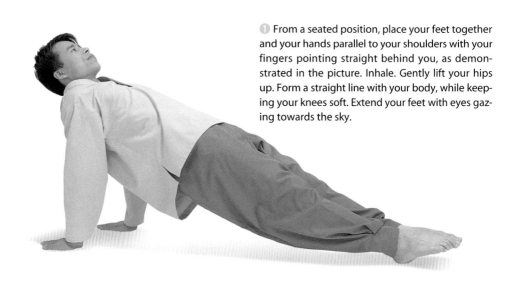

❶ From a seated position, place your feet together and your hands parallel to your shoulders with your fingers pointing straight behind you, as demonstrated in the picture. Inhale. Gently lift your hips up. Form a straight line with your body, while keeping your knees soft. Extend your feet with eyes gazing towards the sky.

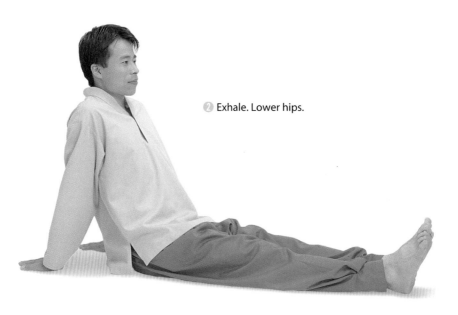

❷ Exhale. Lower hips.

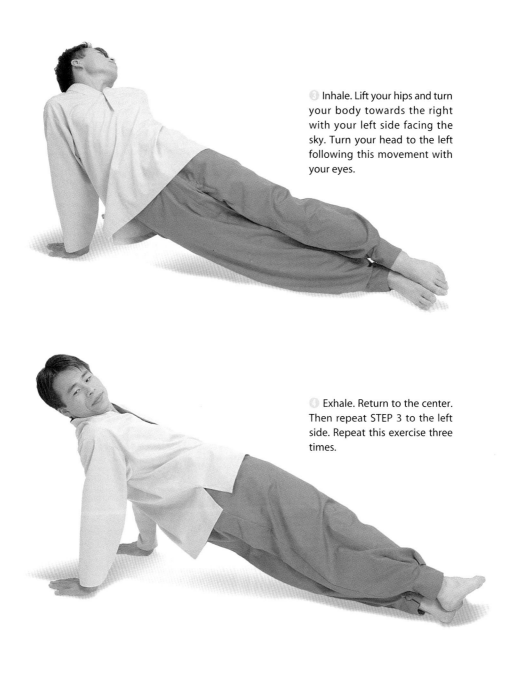

③ Inhale. Lift your hips and turn your body towards the right with your left side facing the sky. Turn your head to the left following this movement with your eyes.

④ Exhale. Return to the center. Then repeat STEP 3 to the left side. Repeat this exercise three times.

2) HYPERTENSION

Symptoms that can signal a problem with hypertension (high blood pressure) include: headaches, anxiety, ringing in the ears, shortness of breath, tightness in the chest, tingling and/or numbness in the legs, nose bleeds, and a possible pulling or sensation of pressure at the back of the neck.

A hallmark in the self-healing treatment for hypertension is to develop the ability to mitigate tension and anxiety through relaxation, meditation and the Dahnhak Meridian exercises recommended in this chapter. Through this practice, blood vessels, which become constricted with the condition of hypertension, can begin to relax. Breathing and meditation exercises are best accomplished in a lying down position. When performing the Dahnhak Meridian exercises, breathe naturally and do not hold your breath. Also headstands are not recommended because blood can rush to the brain quickly and exacerbate the hypertension. As you progress in the Meridian exercises, you can experience sweating and increased warmth in the body as the blood vessels lessen their constriction and begin to open.

BODY TAPPING (Book 1, p. 22)

Benefits Releases stagnant energy throughout the body. Enhances blood and Ki energy circulation.

TIPS Beginners are cautioned to pat gently and comfortably. As you progress, the patting can be applied with more pressure.

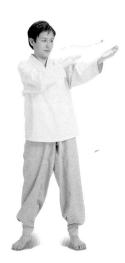

CIRCULATION EXERCISE (Book 1, p. 26)

Benefits Releases stagnant energy that has accumulated in the body. Enhances peripheral blood circulation to the heart thereby lowering blood pressure.

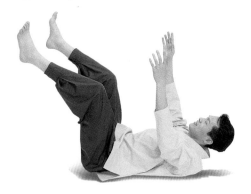

1. STIMULATING PALMS AND SOLES

Benefits The palms of the hands and the soles of the feet are connected to the respiratory and circulatory system and their adjacent organs. Through massaging, or patting and clapping to stimulate the hands and feet, blood and Ki energy circulation is enhanced and the clearing of the mind is accelerated. This is helpful in relieving the symptoms of hypertension or hypotension.

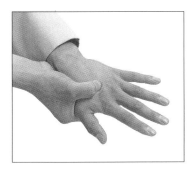 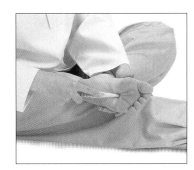

When you stimulate your palms, first locate the Jang-shim acupressure points in your palms. Then turn your hand and touch the spot opposite the Jang-shim. Press with your thumb as shown in the picture and begin to massage. This is located approximately between the index and middle finger.

For the soles of the feet, make a fist and pat or hit your feet. Locate the Yong-chun acupressure points in the soles of your feet, and press with your thumb. You can also use a wooden acupressure point stick. Do this at least ten minutes a day.

BREATHING WHILE WALKING

Exercise is necessary for the treatment of hypertension. However, strenuous exercise can be deleterious. Plan to walk early in the morning for maximum benefit. Breathe in fresh air. Inhale and take three steps. Exhale and take three steps. Focus on your Yong-chun acupressure points as you are walking.

NATURAL REMEDIES

Proper fasting with supplemental nutrition in conjunction with guidance from a trained and reputable health care practitioner can assist in the release of stagnant feces in the intestine that accumulates over time, becoming toxic, and often times causing uncomfortable gastrointestinal symptoms such as constipation and other diseases and conditions.

Wind-Bathing: When it is early in the morning, allow the sun and fresh air to enter the room. Cover your naked body with a blanket. Expose your body to the fresh air and sun and then cover your body again with the blanket. Repeat this several times.

3. CONNECTING THE JANG-SHIM AND YONG-CHUN ACUPRESSURE POINTS WITH BREATHING

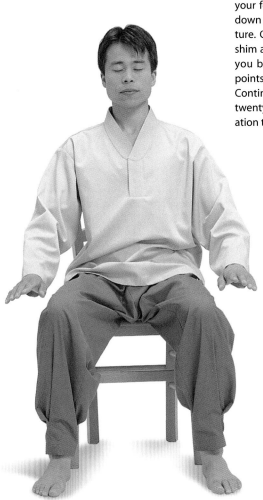

Sit in a chair with your spine straightened and your neck and shoulders relaxed. Place your feet flat on the floor with your palms down and to the sides, as shown in the picture. Close your eyes. Focus on your Jang-shim and Yong-chun acupressure points as you breathe. Imagine these acupressure points as one continuous flow of Ki energy. Continue to breathe like this for fifteen to twenty minutes. Notice the increased relaxation throughout your body.

3. DEEP RELAXATION BREATHING

Benefits Relaxation is the most important exercise you can do. With repeated practice, Ki and blood energy circulation is enhanced and activated. Immune function is boosted thereby expediting the self-healing process. Through this exercise, you can become aware of the sensation of the Ki energy flow throughout your body with mindful focus.

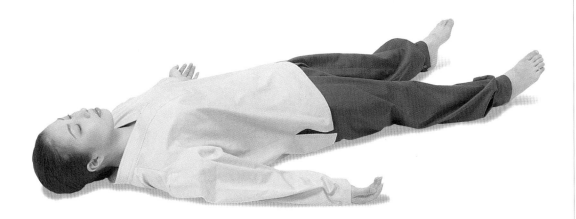

① Lie on your back comfortably as shown in the picture. Scan your body and imagine it as a block of ice with the warm sun radiating upon it. Imagine the warm rays of the sun melting the ice first at the top of your head, then the forehead, face, throat, neck, back, chest, back, hip joints, buttocks, back and front of your thighs, legs, feet, toes, shoulders, arms, hands and fingers. Imagine your body becoming a flowing stream of water. Scan your body for any part that needs further melting and focus on it until you experience it transforming into flowing water.

② Relax your whole body. Begin to become increasingly more relaxed and comfortable. Notice your breath becoming deeper and slower. Focus on your heart. Feel the warmth. Repeat three times: My mind is becoming more and more comfortable.

③ Imagine warm energy flowing from the Im-maek(see page 187) to your Dahn-jon. Continue breathing comfortably, becoming more and more relaxed.

4. PRESSING THE ACUPRESSURE POINTS FOR HYPERTENSION

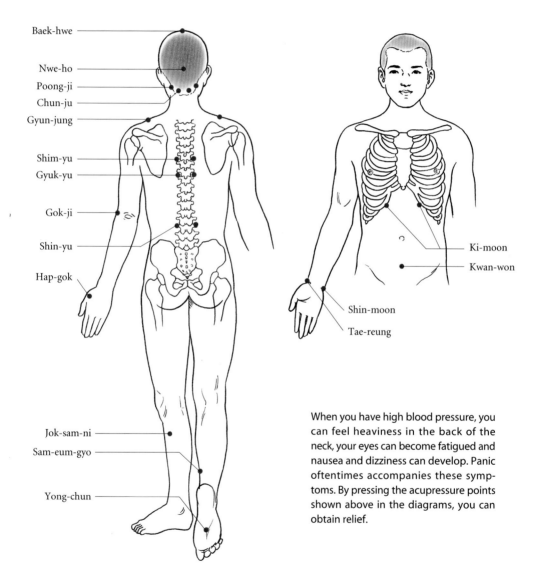

Baek-hwe

Nwe-ho
Poong-ji
Chun-ju
Gyun-jung

Shim-yu
Gyuk-yu

Gok-ji

Shin-yu

Hap-gok

Ki-moon
Kwan-won

Shin-moon
Tae-reung

Jok-sam-ni
Sam-eum-gyo

Yong-chun

When you have high blood pressure, you can feel heaviness in the back of the neck, your eyes can become fatigued and nausea and dizziness can develop. Panic oftentimes accompanies these symptoms. By pressing the acupressure points shown above in the diagrams, you can obtain relief.

5. STRENGTHENING THE HEART MERIDIAN

Benefits Stimulates the Heart Meridian as it strengthens the small and large intestine.

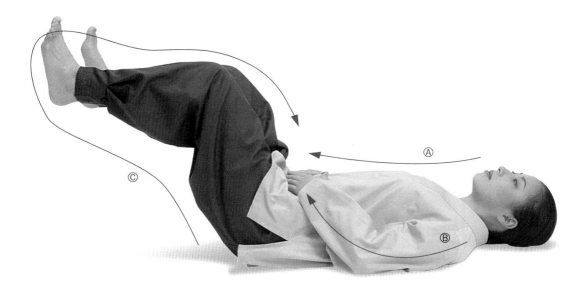

① Lie on your back and assume the posture shown in the picture. Raise your knees and your ankles 90-degrees, while flexing your feet. Relax your neck and shoulders.

② Place both of your hands on your lower abdomen with your thumbs and index fingers touching to form a triangle.

③ Breathe gently and scan the body with your mind's eye in the following progression: A: face, neck, chest, abdomen, Dahn-jon. B: shoulders, arms, Dahn-jon. C: both thighs, legs, toes, Yong-chuns, knees, thighs and Dahn-jon.

④ Focus on your Lower Dahn-jon. Perform Dahn-jon breathing. When you inhale, focus upon the energy coming through the Yong-chun acupressure poinst to the Dahn-jon. When you exhale, focus on the stagnant energy from the Dahn-jon releasing through the toes. If concentrating is difficult for you at this time, go back to STEP 3 and practice by focusing with your mind's eye. Return to Dahn-jon breathing.

3) HYPOTENSION (LOW BLOOD PRESSURE)

The conditions of hypotension and hypertension are both related to the malfunctioning of the blood vessels. symptoms of hypotension include chronic fatigue, dizziness, difficulty with memory and concentration, heart palpitations, tightness or pain in the chest, pale face, weak and slow pulse, and coldness in the hands and feet. Eventually the body functions can be compromised. When you arise suddenly from a sitting position, you may experience dizziness and in the extreme case, you may lose consciousness. When you awake from sleep, you can experience inertia and decreased motivation to participate in life's activities.

These Dahnhak Meridian exercises recommended in this chapter will help ease the symptoms of hypotension. They will assist in enhancing the functioning of the heart in more effectively moving oxygenated blood through the organs and the extremities. When you accompany Meridian exercises with breathing, the effectiveness will be increased. The progression in the performing of these exercises should be gradual in order to be most beneficial for your health and well-being.

SHOULDERSTAND WITH WAIST SUPPORT
(Book 1, p. 96)

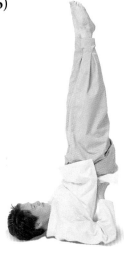

LIFTING THE UPPER BODY
(Book 1, p. 107)

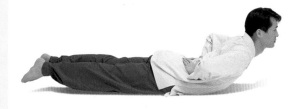

PUSH-UP
(Book 1, p. 137)

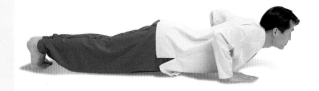

1. WHEELBARROW POSTURE

TIPS   Avoid this exercise if you have hypertension or heart disease

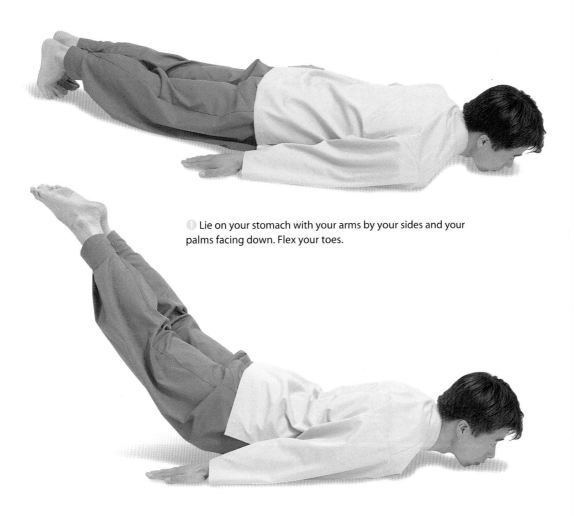

① Lie on your stomach with your arms by your sides and your palms facing down. Flex your toes.

② Inhale. As you hold your breath, put your strength in your Dahn-jon. Push with your hands while lifting both of your legs in the air. Use your Dahn-jon and hands to support you.

③ Hold this position for several seconds or as long as you can, and exhale slowly while bringing your legs down gently. Repeat three times.

2. SQUATS

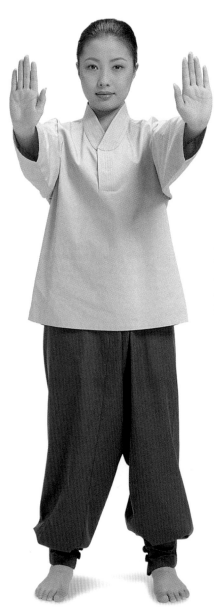

❶ Stand with feet shoulder width apart and your spine straightened. Relax your neck and shoulders. Place both of your arms forward at shoulder level with your hands flexed.

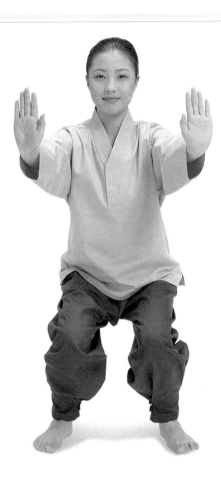

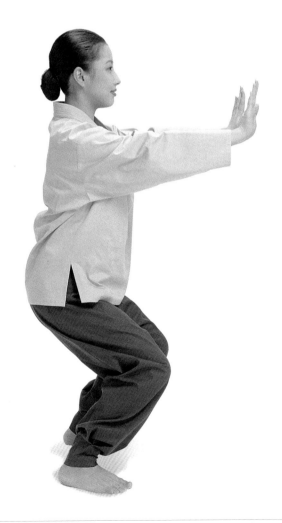

② Lower your body as if preparing to sit. Rise slowly to STEP 1 position. Repeat twenty times.

③ Keep your spine strainght and when bending to sit, keep your knees at a 90-degree angle.

4) STROKE

The human brain houses an intricate vascular webbing and communication system. It is imperative to have continuous blood circulation throughout the brain. If the blood flow becomes restricted in any way, the brain will be deficient of prime nutrients and fresh oxygen. If the situation is such that the continuous blood flow to the brain is blocked or clots, brain tissue can die from the lack of oxygen. This is called ischemic stroke. It is the most commonly occurring of all strokes. The second kind of stroke that can occur is a hemorrhagic stroke. This is when a rupturing of the cerebral artery occurs. This is also known as an aneurysm. There is but another kind of a stroke, called transient ischemic attack (TIA). This is a more benign form of stroke. It is important to discern when this occurs for it can be a warning sign around the occurrence of a more severe form of stroke.

The factors that are associated with a proclivity for stroke include: high blood pressure, diabetes, high cholesterol, irregular heart beat or other heart conditions or disease, smoking and alcohol use, and a history of TIA's. The symptoms that may signal the onset of a stroke include: experiencing numbness in the hands and feet, weakness in facial muscles, usually occurring on one side of the body, insomnia, dizziness, shortness of breath, suddenly occurring severe headache, difficulty with visual acuity, difficulty walking and maintaining coordination and balance, dysarthria (difficulty articulating due to muscle damage to the Peripheral or central nervous system).

The consequential damage from having suffered a stroke can include paralysis or weakness, dysarthria and other language problems, post-stroke depression and emotional lability, pain, and learning and memory deficiencies. It is imperative that prophylactic measures be taken based on current medical knowledge regarding health care, in order to reduce the possibility of a stroke.

The exercises that follow need to be performed with patience if in fact you have experienced a stroke. Keeping your body active is crucial and avoidance of long periods of being sedentary is not recommended. It is helpful to place two walnuts in your hand while moving and rubbing the fingers as you rotate the walnuts to enhance circulation. In addition, Dahnhak Hwal-gong (Acupressure Massage with application of Ki energy) is helpful for post-stroke rehabilitation to enhance energy and blood circulation.

BODY TAPPING (Book 1, p. 22)   **CIRCULATION EXERCISE (Book 1, p. 26)**

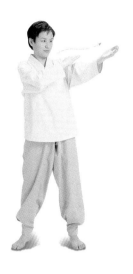
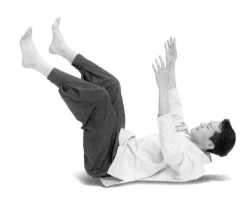

1. HANDS RUBBING

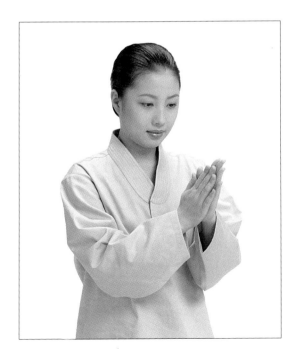

Cup your hands together without touching the Jang-shim acupressure points in the center of the palms. Rub your hands to create heat. Count to ten, and then stop for a few seconds. Rub again and repeat ten times.

2. COMBING HAIR WITH FINGERS

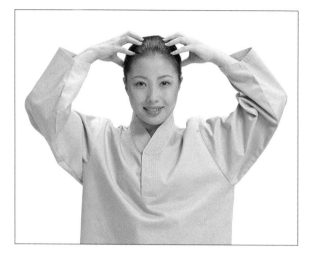

Relax. Spread and bend your fingers. Begin at the forehead and move towards the back of the head and around the circumference of the head. Then press with your fingers all around your head.

PRINCIPLES OF HANG-GONG

Hang-gong exercise is designed to correct and balance mind and body. It restores organs and bones and symmetry. It facilitates Dahn-jon breathing. As your mind focuses on your Dahn-jon, Ki energy circulates throughout the meridians. The accumulation of cosmic Ki energy in the Dahn-jon restores and strengthens the natural healing power of the entire body. With continued practice, you develop confidence in the power, functionality and natural benevolence of your body.

This exercise is practiced with increased intensity over time. It is not meant to perform under pressure or forcefulness in an attempt to maintain the posture with strain. In fact, you may experience adverse effects by doing so. It is therefore recommended that you perform this exercise according to the abilities of your body at the particular time in which you engage in Hang-gong practice.

3. HANG-GONG FOR CIRCULATION
- SUPERMAN POSTURE

Benefits Assists in optimal functioning of the organs and restores body condition through enhanced blood and Ki energy circulation. When there is a deficiency of Ki energy in the body, a stroke can occur. This Hang-gong position will help to accumulate and strengthen Ki energy throughout the body while opening the energy blockages and strengthening the autonomic nervous system.

TIPS Perform this exercise comfortably. Do not force yourself to maintain the posture. With practice you will be able to assume the posture over longer periods of time.

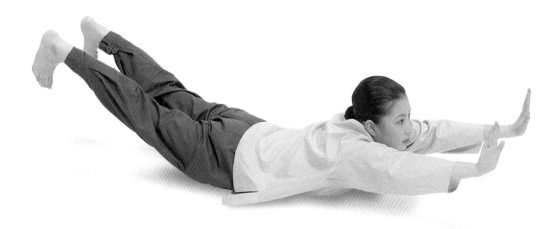

This posture is very difficult, particularly in the initial phases of your learning . With concentration, you will be able to direct and balance Ki energy flow. Observe your body condition and perform daily if you can. If you experience vibration and shaking, this signals releasing of energy blockages. Maintain this posture for about two minutes or less in the beginning, depending on your body condition. With practice you can increase this to thirty minutes or more.

1)GASTROINTESTINAL (GI) DISORDERS

Gastrointestinal (stomach, intestinal) functioning is impacted by emotions and thoughts. It is essential that you practice Dahn-jon breathing to enable the accessing of Alpha brain waves to calm the mind and body. You can consciously control Ki energy with your mind. In order to maximize this, it is helpful to relax your body and mind in the following manner. Close your eyes and scan your body from the top of your head down to your toes with your mind's eye. As you concentrate in this way, you are helping to bring fire energy down to the Dahn-jon.

By performing Dahn-jon breathing your abdomen will become warm and Ki energy surges. Blockages are released and maximal functioning of the stomach and other vital organs can be realized. By practicing consistently, you are attaining the universal principle for both nature and the human body called, Su-Seung-Hwa-Gang, which means water energy up and fire energy down. When the body attains this imperative balance, you will notice the increase of precious saliva in your mouth. As you swallow, this saliva will flow to the lower abdomen and promote healing of the gastrointestinal tract.

JOK-SAM-NI HITTING (Book 1, p.38)

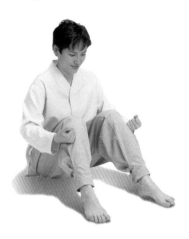

TWISTING AND BENDING THE UPPER BODY WITH LOCKED FINGERS (Book 1, p. 74)

Benefits This exercise eases swelling, bloating, and problems with obesity, regulates appetite control, releases excess fat from abdomen and thighs, helps control diabetes, and realigns lumbar vertebrae and sacrum.

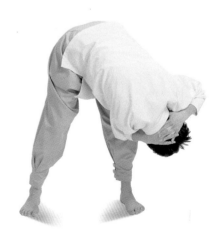

PUSHING WITH ONE HAND ABOVE HEAD
(Book 1 , p. 139)

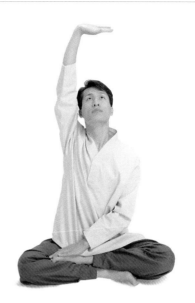

Benefits Stagnant energy from associated energy blocks in the abdomen can be released. Stomach functioning is enhanced.

TIPS Press your left hand on the sole of your foot. As you raise the hand, follow the back of the hand with your eyes.

1. ABDOMINAL BREATHING FOR WEAK STOMACH

Benefits Accumulates heat energy in the lower abdomen and enables more productive digestion.

TIPS Breathe normally and comfortably. Exaggerate the distending and contracting abdominal movements.

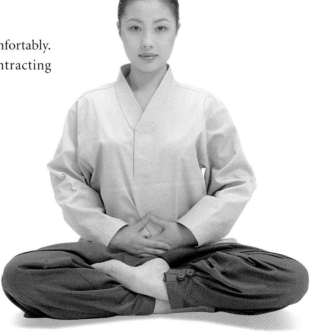

Sit in half lotus position. Place your fingers in a triangle around your Dahn-jon. As you inhale, distend your abdomen as much as possible. As you exhale, contract your abdomen as much as you can. Perform two hundred times.

2. INTESTINE EXERCISES WITH RAISED HIPS

Benefits The Stomach Meridian is stimulated (see page 187- dark blue rectangle). Helps heal GI disorders and strengthen stomach muscles.

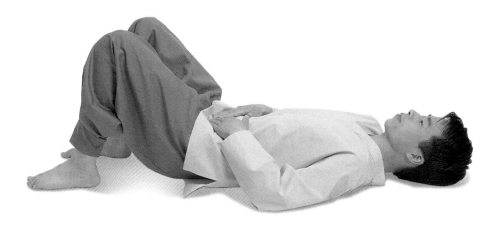

① Lie on your back. Place your legs shoulder width apart and bend your knees with your feet flat on the floor shoulder width apart. Place your hands to form a triangle at the Dahn-jon area.

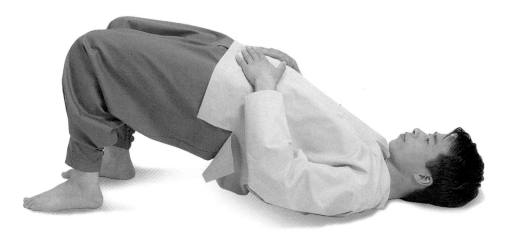

② Lift your hips. Perform intestine exercise by alternating the contraction and the distending of the abdomen. Perform two hundred times. Hold your knees towards center without dropping them to the sides.

3. ARM MASSAGE

Benefits Maximizes Ki energy flow through the arms to strengthen heart, lungs and the GI tract.

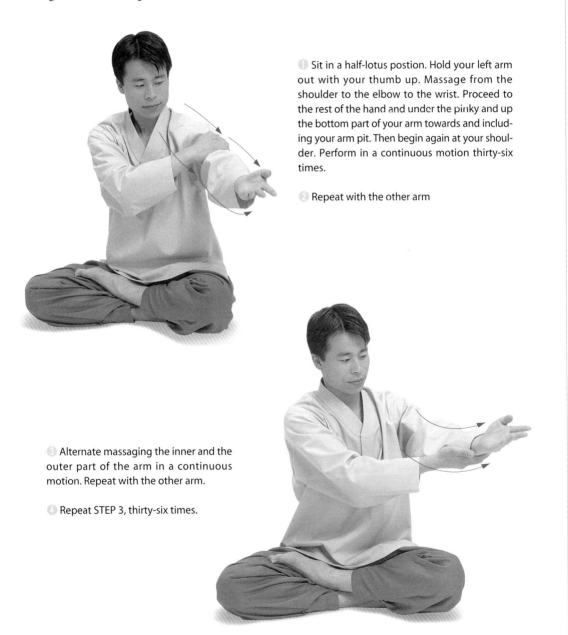

① Sit in a half-lotus postion. Hold your left arm out with your thumb up. Massage from the shoulder to the elbow to the wrist. Proceed to the rest of the hand and under the pinky and up the bottom part of your arm towards and including your arm pit. Then begin again at your shoulder. Perform in a continuous motion thirty-six times.

② Repeat with the other arm

③ Alternate massaging the inner and the outer part of the arm in a continuous motion. Repeat with the other arm.

④ Repeat STEP 3, thirty-six times.

4. FOOT TO THIGH FORWARD BEND

Benefits Accumulated Ki energy in the Dahn-jon is transported to vital organs and the entire body. It helps ulcer healing and balances overproduction of acid secretions in the stomach. This exercise also helps sciatica, numbness in the hands and the feet, helps to relieve shoulder pain, and stimulates appetite.

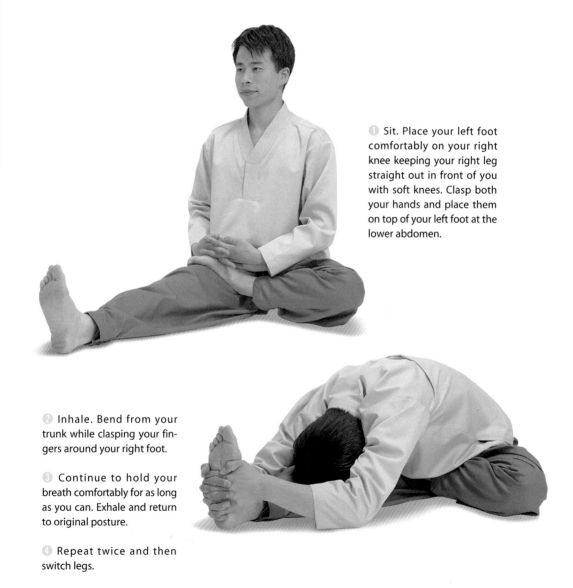

❶ Sit. Place your left foot comfortably on your right knee keeping your right leg straight out in front of you with soft knees. Clasp both your hands and place them on top of your left foot at the lower abdomen.

❷ Inhale. Bend from your trunk while clasping your fingers around your right foot.

❸ Continue to hold your breath comfortably for as long as you can. Exhale and return to original posture.

❹ Repeat twice and then switch legs.

5. ANKLE ROTATION FROM A SEATED POSTURE

Benefits Stimulates the three acupressure points shown in the adjacent picture. Strengthens weak stomach, helps alleviate discomfort from spasms in the stomach.

TIPS When performing this exercise, rotate only the ankle and the foot.

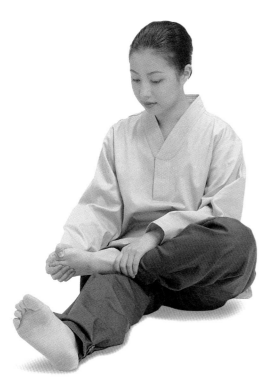

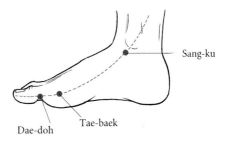

Sang-ku

Tae-baek

Dae-doh

① From a seated posture, extend your right leg with a soft knee and place your left foot on your right knee.

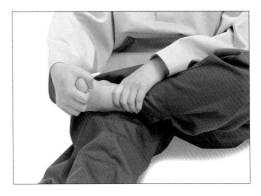

② Hold your left hand on your left ankle gently. With your right hand, flex your toes and alternate flexing and releasing them, four times. Then, with your right hand on your toes, proceed to rotate your ankles clockwise and counter clockwise in wide circles.

6. SITTING SPINAL TWIST

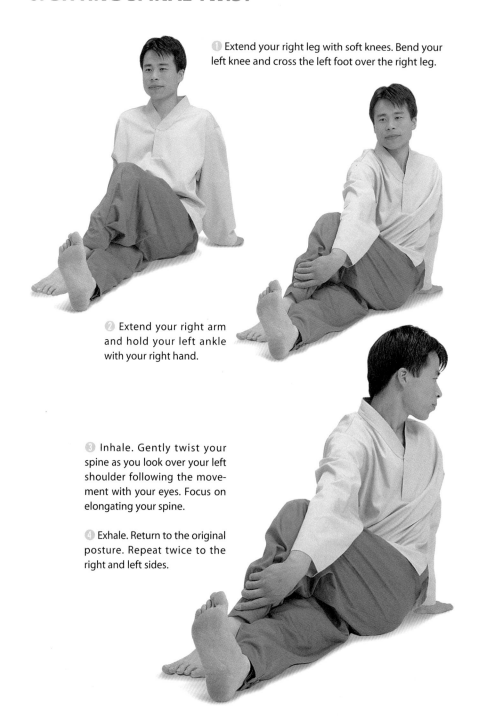

① Extend your right leg with soft knees. Bend your left knee and cross the left foot over the right leg.

② Extend your right arm and hold your left ankle with your right hand.

③ Inhale. Gently twist your spine as you look over your left shoulder following the movement with your eyes. Focus on elongating your spine.

④ Exhale. Return to the original posture. Repeat twice to the right and left sides.

7. ROLLING BACK EXERCISE

Benefits Gently stimulates the spinal cord, strengthens the bone marrow and nervous system, and promotes optimal functioning of the vital organs in the body.

TIPS Let your neck rhythmically follow the motion without pushing with your head. This is best performed on a lightly cushioned surface.

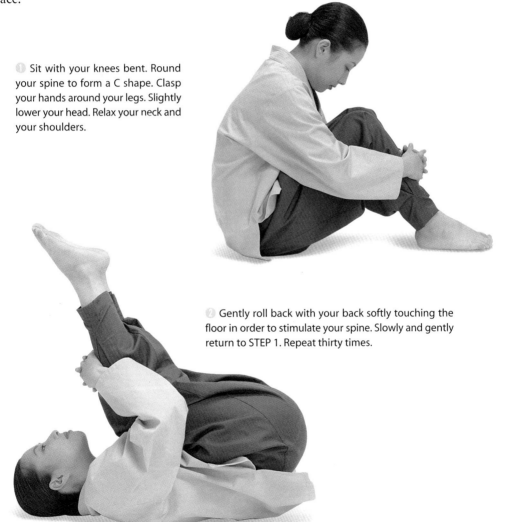

① Sit with your knees bent. Round your spine to form a C shape. Clasp your hands around your legs. Slightly lower your head. Relax your neck and your shoulders.

② Gently roll back with your back softly touching the floor in order to stimulate your spine. Slowly and gently return to STEP 1. Repeat thirty times.

8. UPPER BODY TWIST FROM A PRONE POSTURE

Benefits Stimulates the four acupressure points: Chun-bu, Geuk-chun, Chun-ji and Dae-chu, which strengthens your heart and stomach.

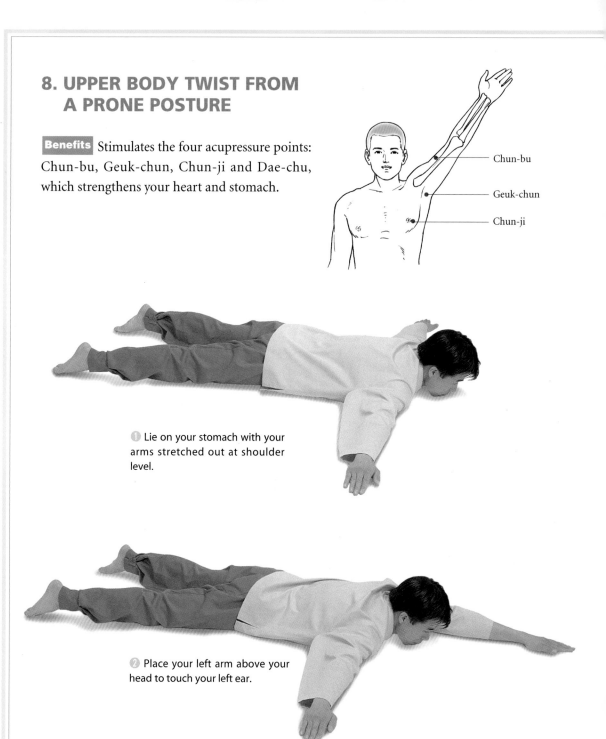

Chun-bu

Geuk-chun

Chun-ji

❶ Lie on your stomach with your arms stretched out at shoulder level.

❷ Place your left arm above your head to touch your left ear.

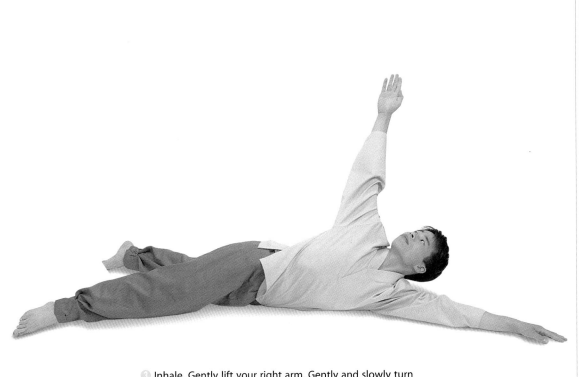

❸ Inhale. Gently lift your right arm. Gently and slowly turn and lift your upper body to the right side while extending your right arm at shoulder level to touch the floor with the palm of your right hand facing up. Keep your legs comfortably still and relax your neck and shoulders. Exhale and slowly return to starting position.

❹ Repeat twice to the right and left sides.

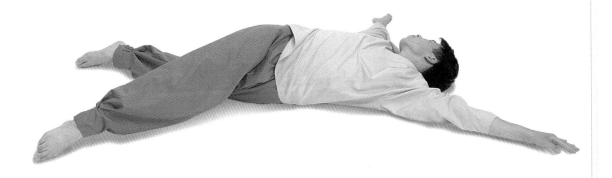

9. HANG-GONG FOR STOMACH

Benefits Stimulates the Stomach Meridian(see page189, # 3) for the GI tract, allowing for healing of the stomach and its associated symptoms of discomfort.

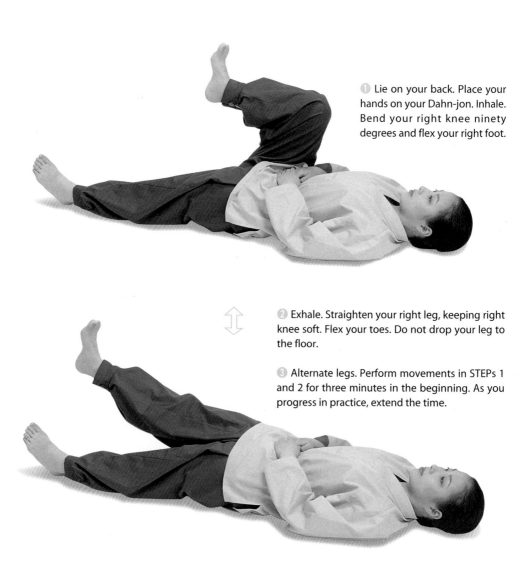

① Lie on your back. Place your hands on your Dahn-jon. Inhale. Bend your right knee ninety degrees and flex your right foot.

② Exhale. Straighten your right leg, keeping right knee soft. Flex your toes. Do not drop your leg to the floor.

③ Alternate legs. Perform movements in STEPs 1 and 2 for three minutes in the beginning. As you progress in practice, extend the time.

10. PRESSING THE UH-JAE ACUPRESSURE POINT

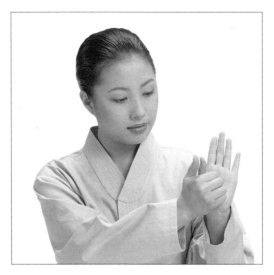

Place your four fingers of one hand on the pad of the palms of the other hand. Press in with your fingers and grasp the pad of the other hand. Continue to press and release. Repeat with your other hand.

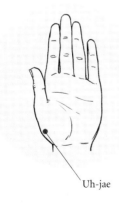

Uh-jae

When you are very fatigued, your body becomes weak and your immune system can become compromised. The condition of the pad of the hand can signal pneumonia or bronchitis. The pad of the hand can feel hot to the touch. Examination of the pads can also signal problems with your other vital organs and discern various symptoms that may be present in the GI tract, such as diarrhea or other conditions of GI imbalance. Performing this exercise can assist in alleviating these symptoms.

2) LIVER DISORDERS

The liver is the largest organ in the body. It fil-ters and cleans the blood and is considered a fat burning organ. As toxicity builds up in the body, liver function is compromised. The predominant symptoms that occur include: tightness in the chest, digestive problems, headaches, depression, dizziness, pain in the joints, sleeping disorders, dry skin/eczema, pallid and tired looking skin, edema, redness in the palms of the hands and tips of the fingers, lethargy, nausea, fatigue, abdominal pain in the upper right quadrant,and difficulty in anger and irritability management. Heat energy remaining in the liver occurs when the anger is not properly negotiated or released from the body. Resultant damage to the liver can occur.

When you perform the exercises recommended, the Liver Meridian becomes stimulated. The body will become warm and the blood and Ki energy will become oxygenated and shunted to the vital organs and the whole body. Increased sweating with these exercises will release toxins. When you breath with your Dahn-jon, the lower abdominal movements synchronize with the movement of the diaphragm, which in turn, stimulates the liver function and the proper circulation of heat ener-gy, thereby enhancing the condition of the liver and trelieving the burden on the liver.

BACK BEND FOR OPENING THE CHEST (Book 1, p. 51)

Benefits Stimulates the thyroid, kidney, liver and pancreas

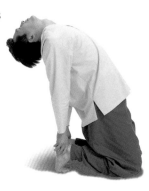

LIFTING LEGS OVER HEAD (Book 1, p 64)

Benefits Stimulates autonomic nervous system and vital organs such as the heart, liver and spleen.

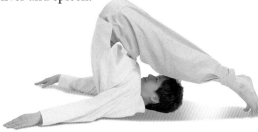

REALIGNING PELVIS AND WAIST (Book 1, p. 102)

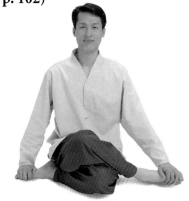

1. EXPANDING CHEST WITH ARM RAISING

TIPS   Keep legs straight with soft knees. Focus on opening your chest.

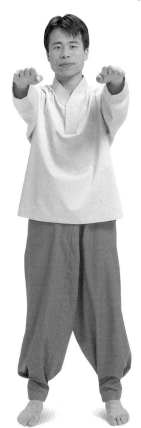

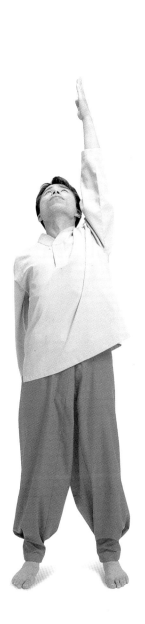

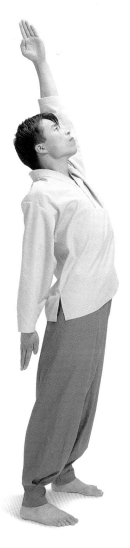

1 Extend arms parallel to the floor with your palms down. Relax your neck and shoulders.

2 Inhale. Raise your left arm up slowly with your palm facing inside. Simultaneously extend your right arm alongside your thigh, hip, and beyond your body with fingers together and thumb facing in the direction of your toes, as shown in the picture. Follow the movement of the arm that is raised with your eyes. Focus upon expansion of your chest.

3 Exhale. Return to STEP 1.

4 Alternate arms. Repeat three times.

2. KNEE RASING WITH FLEXED WRISTS

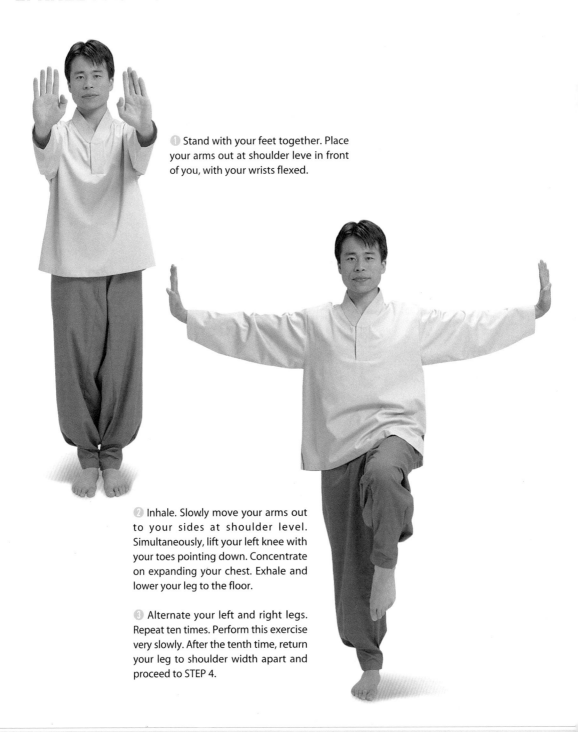

① Stand with your feet together. Place your arms out at shoulder leve in front of you, with your wrists flexed.

② Inhale. Slowly move your arms out to your sides at shoulder level. Simultaneously, lift your left knee with your toes pointing down. Concentrate on expanding your chest. Exhale and lower your leg to the floor.

③ Alternate your left and right legs. Repeat ten times. Perform this exercise very slowly. After the tenth time, return your leg to shoulder width apart and proceed to STEP 4.

3. SIDE BEND WITH FLEXED WRIST

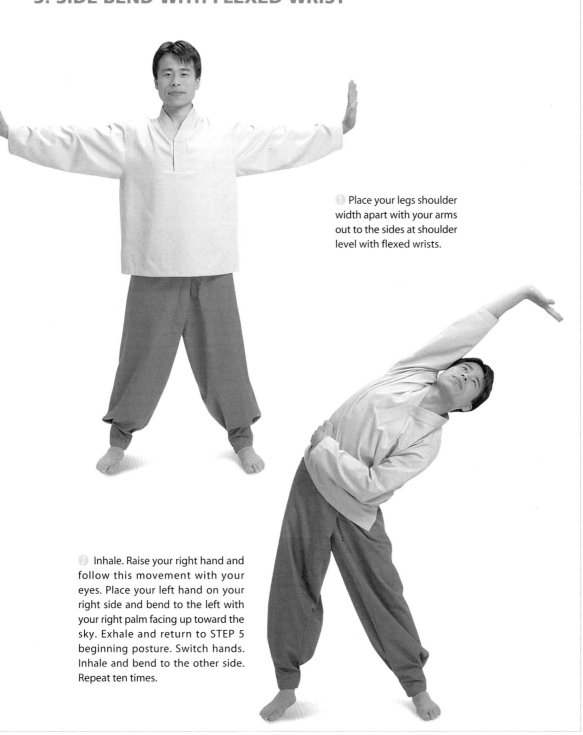

① Place your legs shoulder width apart with your arms out to the sides at shoulder level with flexed wrists.

② Inhale. Raise your right hand and follow this movement with your eyes. Place your left hand on your right side and bend to the left with your right palm facing up toward the sky. Exhale and return to STEP 5 beginning posture. Switch hands. Inhale and bend to the other side. Repeat ten times.

4. LENGTHENING THE NECK

Benefits Releases stagnant energy from the shoulders, chest and arms. Strengthens the lungs and liver.

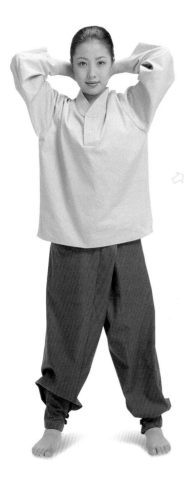

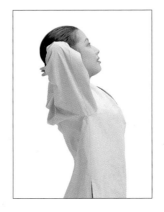

② While continuing to hold your breath and lifting and supporting your neck, tilt your head back. Look at the sky. Focus upon your ribs and spine. Exhale and return to STEP 1.

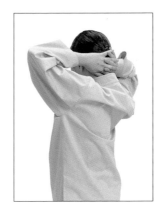

① Inhale. Lock your fingers behind your neck. With both hands, press the back of the neck. Lift and support the back of your neck.

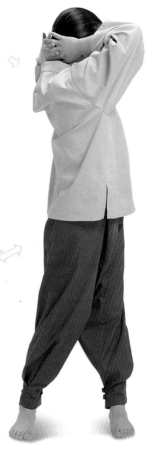

③ Turn to the left and right very slowly ten times.

5. CLAM SHELL SIT-UP

Benefits Enhances liver function in a short period of time.

TIPS Keep your legs and toes straight but with soft knees.

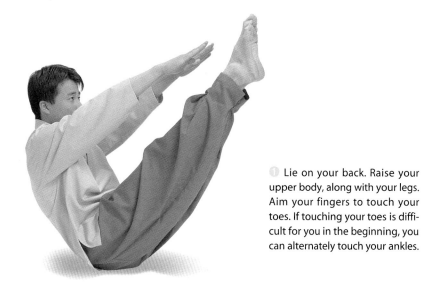

① Lie on your back. Raise your upper body, along with your legs. Aim your fingers to touch your toes. If touching your toes is difficult for you in the beginning, you can alternately touch your ankles.

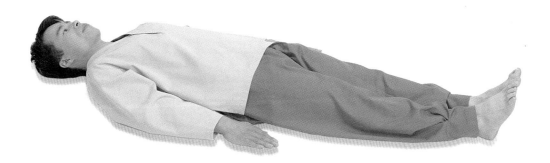

② Return to starting position and relax for ten seconds. Repeat five times.

6. TWISTING KNEES TO TOUCH THE FLOOR

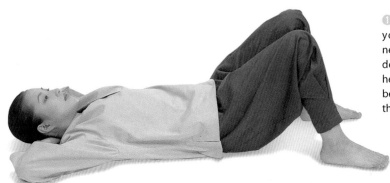

❶ Lie on your back. Lock your fingers behind your neck. Place your legs shoulder width apart. Bring your heels towards your hips and bend your knees as shown in the picture.

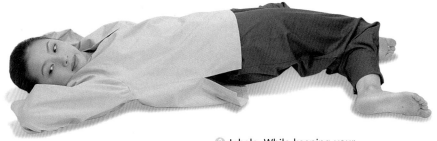

❷ Inhale. While keeping your shoulders still, turn your head to the right side and simultaneously move both knees to the left to touch the floor.

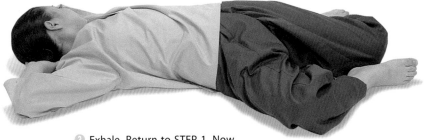

❸ Exhale. Return to STEP 1. Now turn your head to the left side, while simultaneously moving both knees to the right side and touching the floor. Repeat three times, alternating to the left and right sides.

7. SIDE BEND

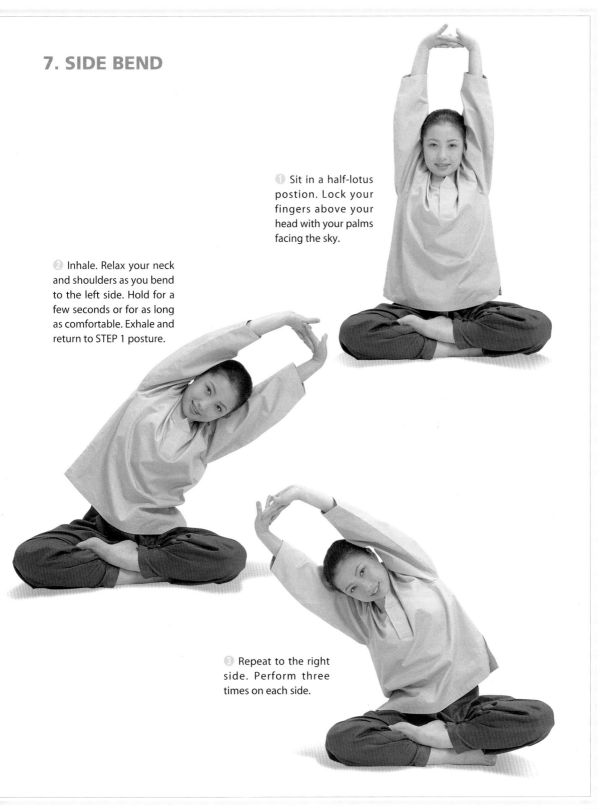

① Sit in a half-lotus postion. Lock your fingers above your head with your palms facing the sky.

② Inhale. Relax your neck and shoulders as you bend to the left side. Hold for a few seconds or for as long as comfortable. Exhale and return to STEP 1 posture.

③ Repeat to the right side. Perform three times on each side.

8. BRIDGE POSTURE

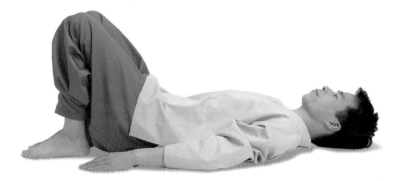

① Lie on your back. Bend your knees. Place your heels together close to your hips.

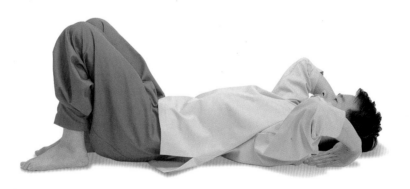

② Place your hands on either side of your head with your fingers pointing towards your feet.

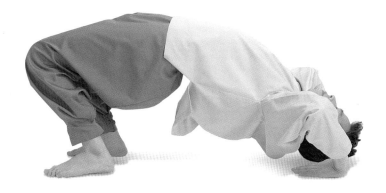

Inhale. Press your hands and feet into the floor while simultaneously raising your shoulders and hips and then your head very comfortably and without strain.

Hold this posture for a few seconds or for as long as you are comfortable.

Relax and exhale. Return to STEP 2 posture. Repeat three times.

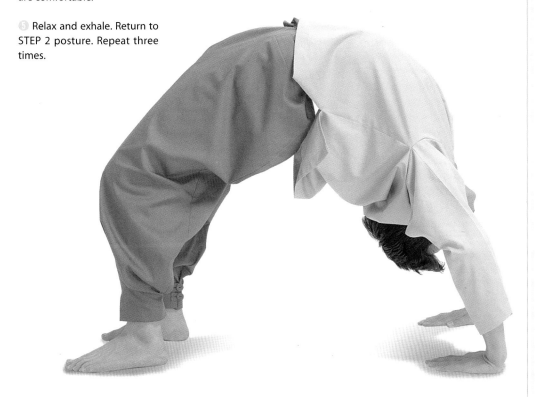

9. CROSSING LEG TO TOUCH FINGERS

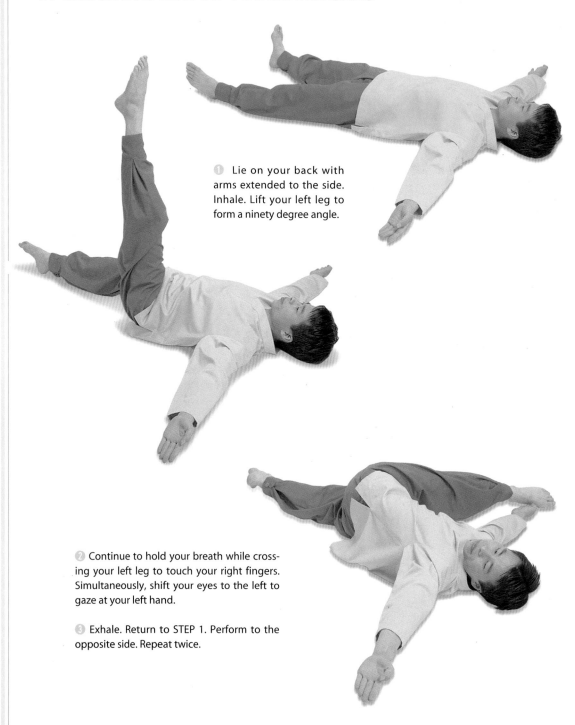

❶ Lie on your back with arms extended to the side. Inhale. Lift your left leg to form a ninety degree angle.

❷ Continue to hold your breath while crossing your left leg to touch your right fingers. Simultaneously, shift your eyes to the left to gaze at your left hand.

❸ Exhale. Return to STEP 1. Perform to the opposite side. Repeat twice.

10. SENDING KI ENERGY TO EYES

Benefits The condition of the eyes can be related to the functioning of the liver. With this exercise, liver conditions can be improved.

TIPS Keep your eyes open during this exercise.

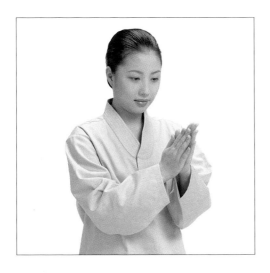

① Inhale deeply through the Dahn-jon. Rub your palms together fifty times.

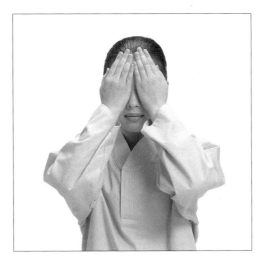

② Place both of your hands over your eyes with the Jang-shim acupressure points closest to your eyes.

③ Exhale. Rotate your eyeballs up and down, clockwise and counterclockwise, and to either side ten times each.

11. TWISTING SIDE TO SIDE WITH LEGS RAISED

TIPS If you have back problems, proceed with caution with this exercise. If you experience any pressure in the head while your legs are raised to a 90-degree angle, you may want to elevate your head very slightly while performing this exercise.

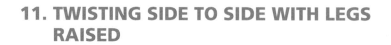

① Lie on your back with your arms extended at shoulder level. Keep your legs together with soft knees, while raising them to a 90-degree angle.

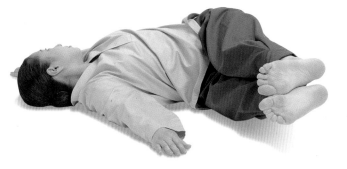

② Inhale. Bring both of your legs to the right and gently touch the floor. Gaze with your eyes in the direction of your left fingers. Hold for about two to three seconds. As you progress in this exercise, you can touch your right hand with your feet. Exhale and slowly brings your legs back to a 90-degree angle as in STEP 1.

③ Lower your feet slowly to the left side while gazing to the right. Repeat five times.

12. TURNING FEET OUT

Benefits This posture will stimulate and strengthen the liver and relieve fatigue. This posture also strengthens the knee joints to prevent arthritis, and strengthens the lower extremities and the Dahn-jon.

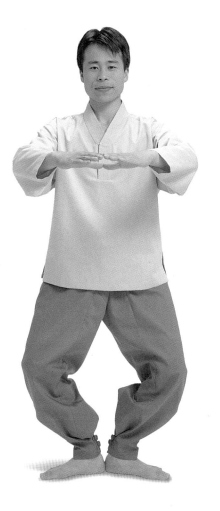

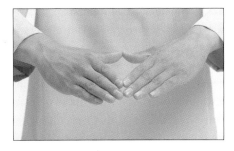

② Form a triangle with your fingers by touching your thumbs and index fingers, with your palms facing down at shoulder level. Relax your neck, shoulders and arms.

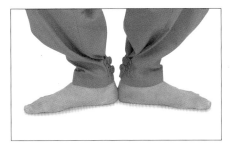

③ Hold this posture for as long as you are comfortable. Accompany this exercise with Dahn-jon breathing as you progress in your practice.

① Stand. Touch your heels together with your feet extended towards a 180-degree angle and your knees bent to a 90-degree angle. Keep your spine straightened with your neck and shoulders relaxed. Place your arms in front of your chest.

3) DIARRHEA

When the large intestine(colon) is functioning properly, it will absorb liquid from the waste frequenting the small intestine. When diarrhea occurs, there is either secretion from the bowel impeding absorption, or the wastes expeditiously pass through the bowel without adequate transit time for the appropriate absorption of fluid.

There are two types of diarrhea: chronic and acute. chronic diarrhea can be related to infection in the intestines or the liver and/or the consumption of foods that produce cold energy, rendering the abdomen cold. Tainted foods can also underlie cases of chronic diarrhea. acute diarrhea is oftentimes related to food poisoning. Symptoms include severe abdominal pain, and repeated episodes of defecation. nausea, headache, and vomiting can accompany these symptoms.

Under normal circumstances, diarrhea can dissipate in two to three days. However, if these aforementioned symptoms persist, particularly accompanied by a high fever and severe pain in the abdomen, then a more serious condition can be present, warranting medical attention. Diarrhea can be generated and exacerbated by the presence of stress and irregular and erratic eating habits. It is helpful to stimulate the feet, palms, and lower abdomen with massage to assist in the improvement of the digestive process and enhance the absorption process.

SITTING FORWARD BEND
(Book 1, p. 52)

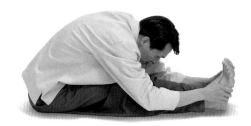

LIFTING LEGS OVER HEAD
(Book 1, p. 64)

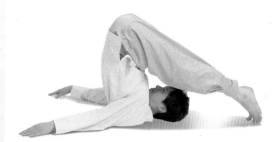

1. PRESSING DAE-JANG-YU ACUPRESSURE POINTS

TIPS   It is important to focus on expanding your chest to relax your body while performing this exercise.

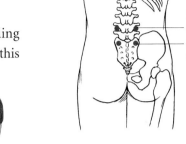

Dae-jang-yu
(for large intestine)

So-jang-yu
(for small intestine)

Dae-jang-yu acupressure points are located about two inches to either side of the Fourth and Fifth Lumbar Vertebrae.The So-jang-yu acupressure points are about one inch below the Dae-jang-yu points.

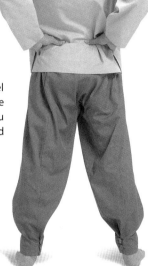

① Stand with your feet parallel and shoulder width apart. Place your thumbs on the Dae-jang-yu acupressure points, as depicted in the diagram.

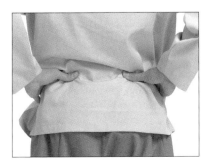

② Inhale. Slowly tilt your upper trunk backwards slightly. Simultaneously press with your thumbs in the Dae-jang-yu points. Contract your anal muscles. Hold for as long as comfortable.

③ Exhale and return to STEP 1.

2. TAPPING THE SO-JANG-YU AND THE DAE-JANG-YU ACUPRESSURE POINTS

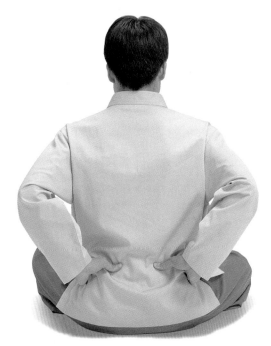

❶ Sit in a half-lotus postion. Place and press your thumbs on the So-jang-yu acupressure points.

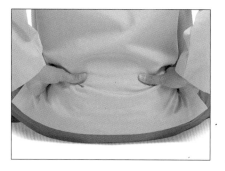
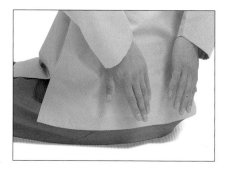

❷ Pat the So-jang-yu points until you generate heat energy in this area. Follow with rubbing in the vicinity of these acupressure points with a quick motion.

❸ Repeat STEPs 1 and 2 with the Dae-jang-yu points.

3. WAIST LIFTING

Benefits Stops mild diarrhea.

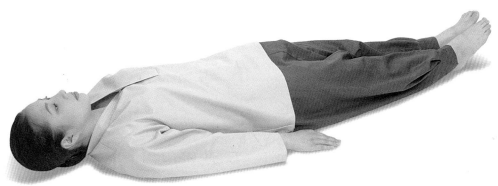

① Lie on your back with your feet together with your hands by your side.

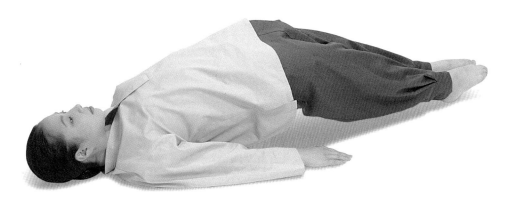

② Inhale. Raise your waist, hips and back gently and slowly. Support your body with your hands, arms and your heels remaining on the floor while lifting.

③ Hold this posture for ten seconds. Exhale and lower your body gently to the floor. Repeat five times.

4) CONSTIPATION

✿

There are three main factors in the etiology of constipation: stress, age and hormones. Constipation occurs and toxins begin to accumulate over time, spreading throughout the body and incubating disease. Aging can become accelerated, cerebral vascular functioning can become adversely affected, and gastro-intestinal tract disturbances increase in severity, as could headaches, high blood pressure, and the eruption of skin disorders.

Seniors are particularly vulnerable to a proclivity for constipation. As one ages, the peristaltic movements are not as efficient. Waste products accumulate in the intestine for a prolonged period of time. Water and moisture become absorbed, precluding the ability to efficiently transit the fecal waste material to exit the body. It is imperative to exercise and particularly to maintain and strengthen abdominal muscles. Women also develop constipation with more frequency. Hormonal changes in the menstrual cycle impact the secretion of hormones that compress the peristaltic motions of the large intestine.

When you perform these Meridian exercises, it is imperative to accompany them with Dahn-jon breathing with mindfulness on the coordination of the breath and synchronous movements of expanding and contracting the abdomen for maximized benefit.

INTESTINAL EXERCISE (Book 1, p. 28)

TIPS Concentrate on expansion and contraction of the lower abdomen as much as you can.

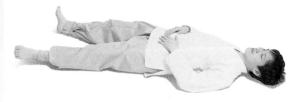

SIT-UP (Book 1, p. 108)

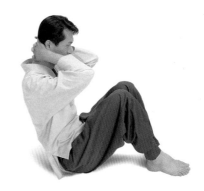

TAILBONE TAPPING (Book 2, p .125)

Benefits Enhances the autonomic nervous system and efficient peristaltic movements.

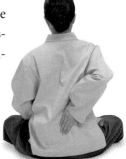

1. FISH EXERCISE

Benefits Strengthens spinal nerves and enriches blood circulation. Keeps the intestines in their proper placement and shape, and relieves constipation.

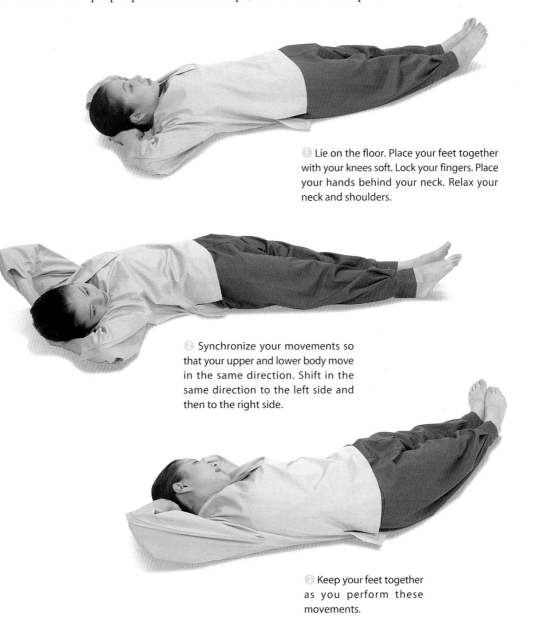

① Lie on the floor. Place your feet together with your knees soft. Lock your fingers. Place your hands behind your neck. Relax your neck and shoulders.

② Synchronize your movements so that your upper and lower body move in the same direction. Shift in the same direction to the left side and then to the right side.

③ Keep your feet together as you perform these movements.

2. LEG LIFT VARIATION

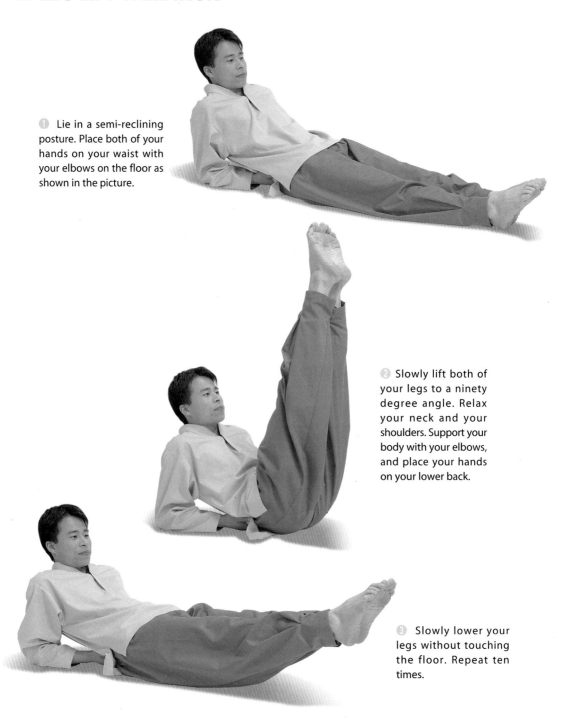

① Lie in a semi-reclining posture. Place both of your hands on your waist with your elbows on the floor as shown in the picture.

② Slowly lift both of your legs to a ninety degree angle. Relax your neck and your shoulders. Support your body with your elbows, and place your hands on your lower back.

③ Slowly lower your legs without touching the floor. Repeat ten times.

3. LYING KNEE PULL

Benefits Relieves constipation. Strengthens women's reproductive system.

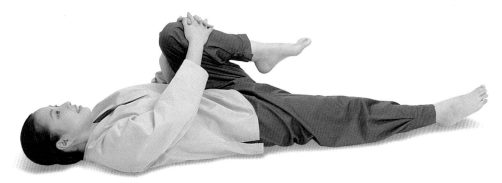

① Lie on your back. Bend your left knee towards your chest. Lock your fingers and grasp the shin of your left leg. Extend your right leg straight in front of you maintaining a soft knee.

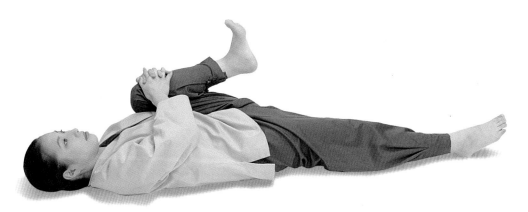

② Inhale. Flex your left foot. Pull your left knee as close to your chest as you can.

③ Exhale. Return to STEP 1. Change legs and proceed as in STEPs 1 through 3. Repeat three times with each leg.

4. CONTRACTING AND EXPANDING DAHN-JON

① Lie on your back. Lock your fingers around the shins of your legs with your knees bent.

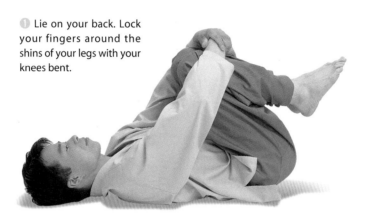

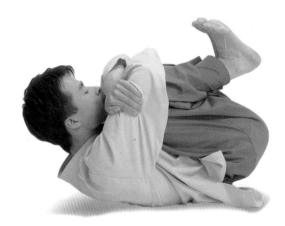

② Inhale. Gently crunch your body as you pull your knees to your chest, while simultaneously gently lifting your head to touch your knees. Focus on your Dahn-jon.

③ Exhale. Slowly and gently lower your legs and place your feet on the floor, with your knees bent. Bring your arms by your side with your palms facing the floor. Relax your body.

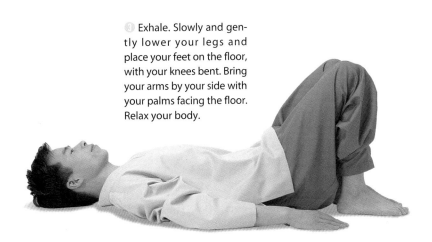

④ Inhale. Gently lift your lower abdomen to the sky as much as you comfortably can. Exhale to STEP 3. Repeat three times.

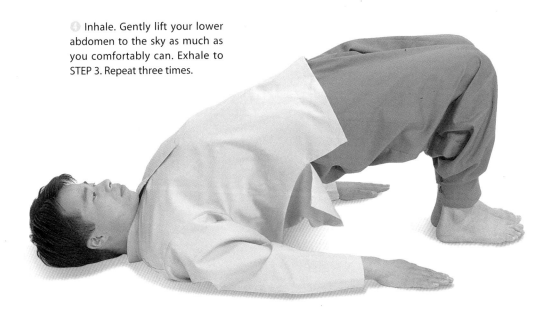

5. BOW POSTURE WITH ROLLING

Benefits Realigns the spine and strengthens peristaltic movement of the intestines thereby healing problems with constipation. Releases toxins as it aids the elimination process.

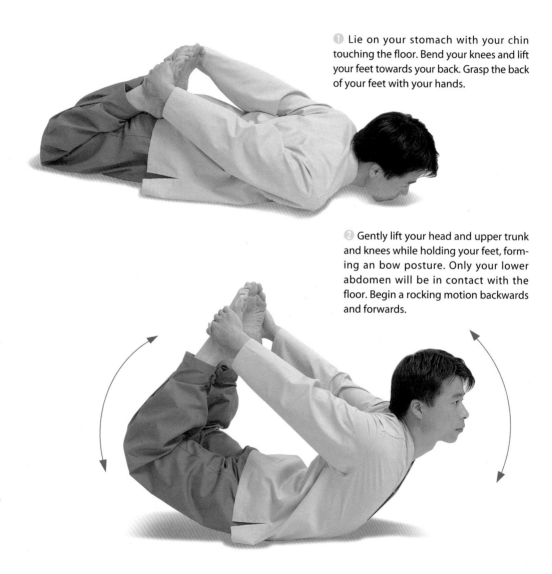

① Lie on your stomach with your chin touching the floor. Bend your knees and lift your feet towards your back. Grasp the back of your feet with your hands.

② Gently lift your head and upper trunk and knees while holding your feet, forming an bow posture. Only your lower abdomen will be in contact with the floor. Begin a rocking motion backwards and forwards.

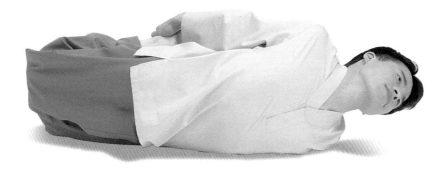

③ Gently turn to your left side and rock gently
to the right and to the left. Gently turn to your
right side and engage the rocking motion to the
right and to the left.

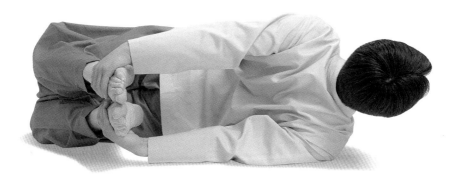

④ Repeat the above steps, but this time, perform your motions very slowly, comfortably, and
gently to properly stimulate your organs.

6. WAIST BENDING AND SOLE HITTING

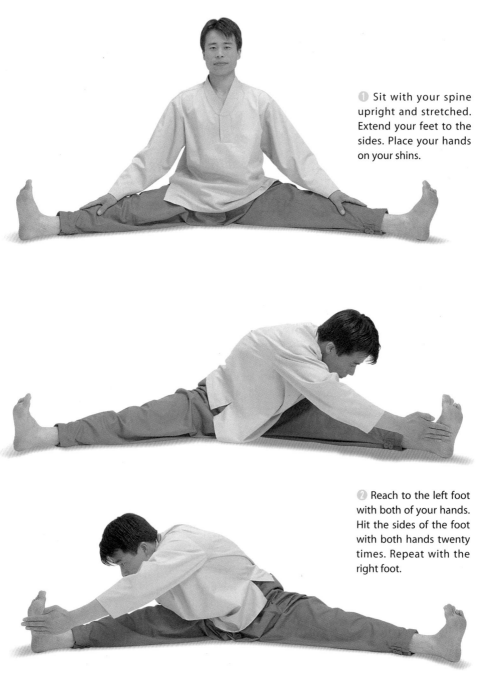

① Sit with your spine upright and stretched. Extend your feet to the sides. Place your hands on your shins.

② Reach to the left foot with both of your hands. Hit the sides of the foot with both hands twenty times. Repeat with the right foot.

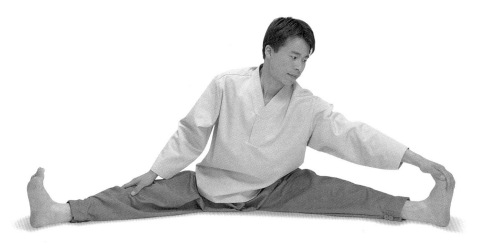

③ Place your left hand on your left toes and your right hand on your right thigh. Bend from the waist while bringing your right hand over to the left foot. Glide your left hand to the back of the foot while placing your right hand around the toes of the left foot. Hold for as long as comfortable while focusing on the bending of your waist.

④ Proceed with exercise on the right side. Repeat on each side.

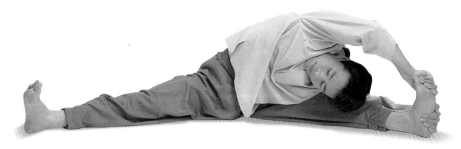

5) HEMORRHOIDS

Hemorrhoids occur when the blood vessels around the circumference of the anus become swollen. This is due to the accumulation of the pooling of stagnant blood in the anal area. When you sit or stand for a long time, maintaining the same posture, there is increased pressure around the anus. If you suffer from constipation, the problem is exacerbated under the extreme pressure that occurs. It is important to maintain warmth in the lower abdomen, take measures that will ensure healthy elimination patterns, and avoid sitting on a cold surface. There is an association between the proclivity for suffering from hemorrhoids and faulty intestinal functioning. Even in circumstances where one undergoes a hemorrhoidectomy, that person can still suffer from a re-occurrence of the development of hemorrhoids if the problem of the intestines is not explored and resolved.

The exercises recommended will augment healthy shunting of blood flow to the anal area thereby mitigating the swelling of the anal area that causes hemorrhoids to develop. Practicing these Meridian exercises will strengthen the intestines as well as help with the problems associated with constipation.

ANAL CONTRACTING EXERCISE (Book 1, p. 29)

Prevents hemorrhoid formation and treats hemorrhoids when they occur. Eliminates anal swelling by enhancing Ki and blood circulation around the anus. You can practice this exercise anywhere and anyplace.

BICYCLING EXERCISE (Book 1, p. 142)

Strengthens lower extremities, muscles and nerves around the perineum, and reproductive glands. Strengthens Ki and blood circulation. Prevents and treats hemorrhoids. Releases fatigue from the head and the lower extremities as it enhances stamina.

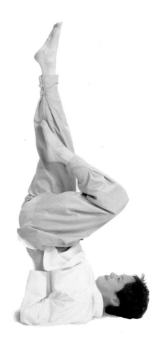

1. TAPPING THE BAEK-HWE ACUPRESSURE POINT

Benefits By pressing on the Baek-hwe acupressure point(top of the head), pain can be alleviated. The Baek-hwe is an acupressure point in the treatment of hemorrhoids.

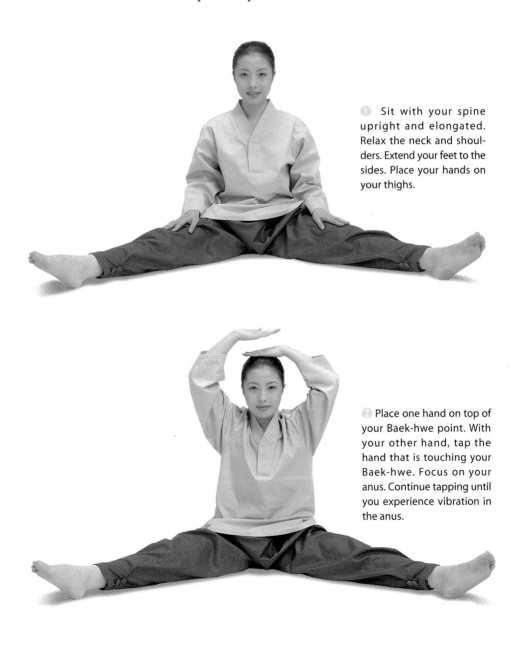

❶ Sit with your spine upright and elongated. Relax the neck and shoulders. Extend your feet to the sides. Place your hands on your thighs.

❷ Place one hand on top of your Baek-hwe point. With your other hand, tap the hand that is touching your Baek-hwe. Focus on your anus. Continue tapping until you experience vibration in the anus.

2. HOLDING ANKLES WHILE LIFTING DAHN-JON

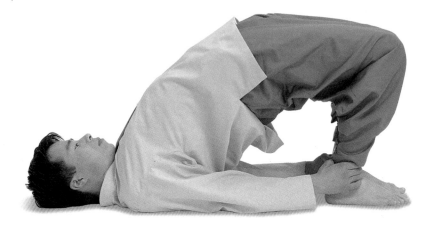

① Lie on your back. Inhale. Gently lift your hips up. Hold this posture while contracting your anus. Focus on your Dahn-jon.

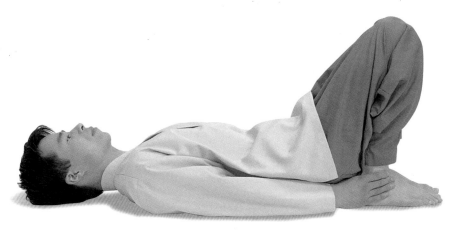

② Exhale. Slowly lower your hips. Repeat five times.

3. STANDING KNEE PULL

① Stand with your feet together. strengthen your spine. Inhale. Lock your fingers and pull your knee towards your chest.

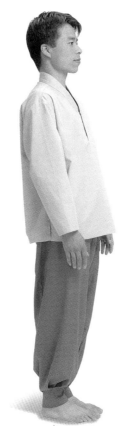

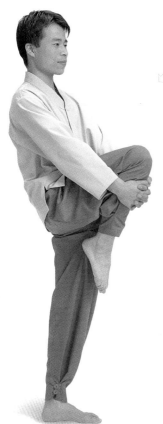

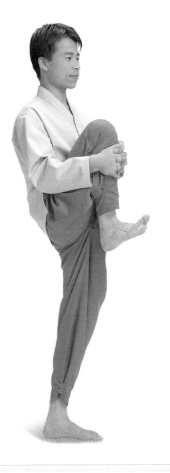

② Flex your foot so your toes face towards the sky. Align your neck and back.

③ Exhale. Unlock your fingers. Return to standing position with both of your feet on the floor. Repeat the above steps with your other leg. Perform three times with each leg.

1) KIDNEY DISORDERS

When there is kidney malfunction, a person can notice edema in the abdomen, legs, a feeling of heaviness in the body, and cold sweats during sleeping hours. There is usually a preference to sleep on your stomach. Upon awakening, you can experience swelling and discomfort around the circumference of your waist.

Medical research has demonstrated that when you perform Dahn-jon breathing, the kidney moves about one to two inches as it is stimulated and massaged in this process, facilitating Ki and blood circulation to this organ.

The kidney is contolling the Jung energy, vital energy in the lower Dahn-jon. It is here where we can observe the kidney and its importance. As you focus your attention on your Myung-moon (the opposite side of the naval) accupressure point, and breathe through this point as part of Dahn-jon breathing, it will lead to the strengthening of the Jung energy in the lower Dahn-jon. As you continue to practice this breathing, the kidney is less burdened in the performance of its job in filtering the blood and excreting toxins from the body. The recommended Meridian exercises in this chapter will stimulate the Bladder Meridian and enhance the functioning of the kidneys.

CIRCULATION EXERCISE
(Book 1, p. 26)

TIPS Extend knees, arms and elbows. If your neck is in discomfort, you may place a wooden pillow under it for support.

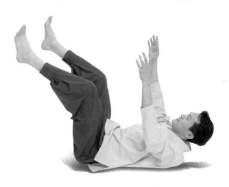

UPPER BODY LIFT
(Book 1, p. 50)

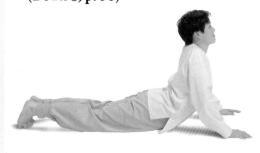

SITTING FORWARD BEND
(Book 1, p. 52)

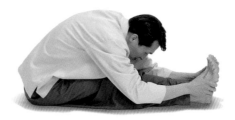

LIFTING LEGS OVER HEAD (Book 1, p. 64)

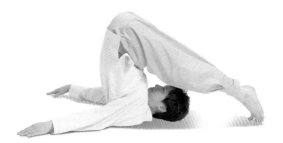

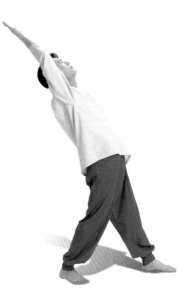

RAISING HANDS (Book 1, p. 71)

TIPS As you tilt backwards, follow the movement with the gaze of your eyes as your arms touch your ears. If you experience dizziness, or if your body condition is weak or you are an elder, minimize your tilting. Gaze with your eyes towards the horizon, rather than towards your fingertips. Place your weight on the back of the right foot, toes, Dahn-jon and waist.

LYING ON YOUR STOMACH WHILE CROSSING LEGS (Book 1, p. 104)

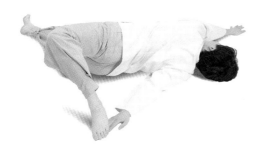

HITTING THE SOLES (Book 1, p. 41; Book 2, p. 16)

Benefits The Yong-chun acupressure points on the soles of the feet are connected to the kidney. It is helpful to practice applying pressure with a wooden stick or your fingers and to stimulate the Yong-chun in the morning for about five minutes.

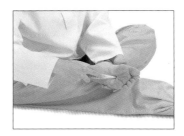

1. PRESSING THE SHIN-YU AND THE JI-SHIL ACUPRESSURE POINTS

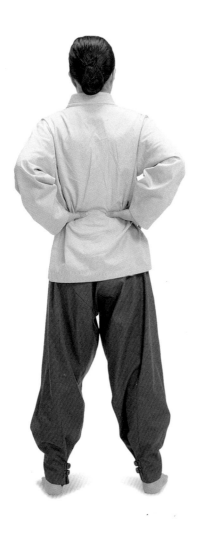

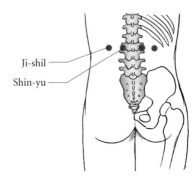

Ji-shil

Shin-yu

- Shin-yu acupressure points are located on either side of the Second Lumbar Vertebrae. In between these two acupressure points is the Myung-moon acupressure point. The Shin-yu points are about one and a half inches on either side at the Myung-moon point. It is located at the Spinal Cord Line Number 1.
- Ji-shil acupressure points are located on either side of the Second Lumbar Vertebrae and about one and one half inches to the outside from the Shin-yu points, and three inches from the Myung-moon. The Ji-shil points are located on Spinal Cord Line Number 2.

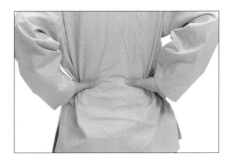

❶ Stand with your feet shoulder width apart. Place your thumbs on the Shin-yu points.

❷ Inhale while you press the Shin-yu points with your thumbs. Gently tilt your upper body backwards.

❸ Continue to hold your breath as you press with your thumbs and focus on your waist.

❹ Release your thumbs. Exhale. Repeat STEPS 1 to 4 twice. Then perform the same exercise with the Ji-shil points.

2. STIMULATING THE KIDNEYS

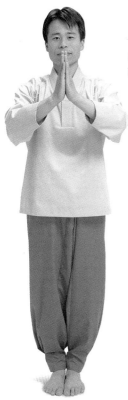

① Stand with your feet together. Place your hands in front of your chest in a prayer position.

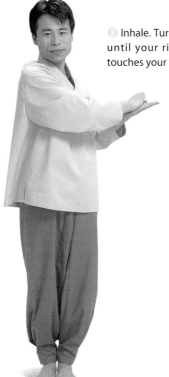

② Inhale. Turn to the left until your right elbow touches your left rib.

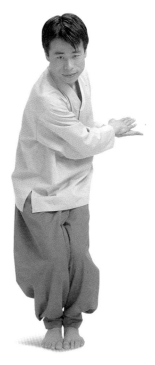

③ Slightly bend your upper body forward while bending your knees. Keep your hands together as well as your feet. Focus on your kidneys.

④ Exhale to Step 1. Repeat to the right side.

3. WHEELBARROW VARIATION

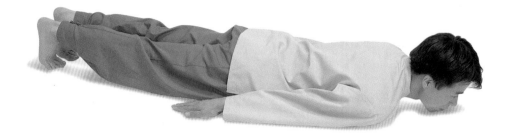

① Lie on your stomach. Place your hands at your sides with palms facing down and toes flexed.

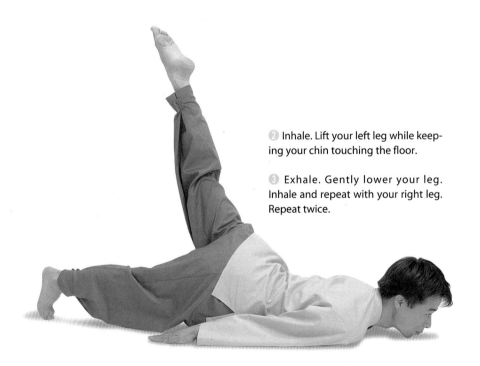

② Inhale. Lift your left leg while keeping your chin touching the floor.

③ Exhale. Gently lower your leg. Inhale and repeat with your right leg. Repeat twice.

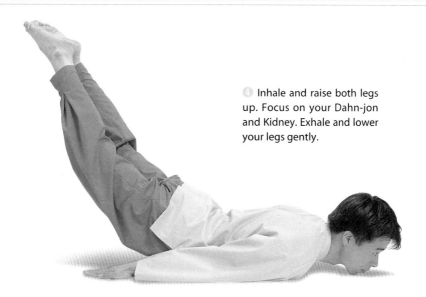

④ Inhale and raise both legs up. Focus on your Dahn-jon and Kidney. Exhale and lower your legs gently.

4. KIDNEY MASSAGE

Benefits Relieves stagnant energy from the kidneys. Allows Ki energy to circulate through the kidneys, which will enhance kidney function. Kidney massage performed directly with your hands to the skin without clothes is beneficial. You can experience coolness throughout the lower extremities.

Inhale. Rub your hands until they are hot. Press your hands on your kidneys with your fingers facing down and massage in an up and down motion.

5. RELEASING ANKLE BLOCKAGES WITH ACUPRESSURE POINTS

Benefits When there is a deficiency of energy in the Dahn-jon, the heel pads can feel rough to the touch, and elasticity in this area begins to decrease. Stimulating the acupressure points shown in the accompanying diagram is helpful. Stamina is enhanced through stimulating the acupressure points demonstrated below.

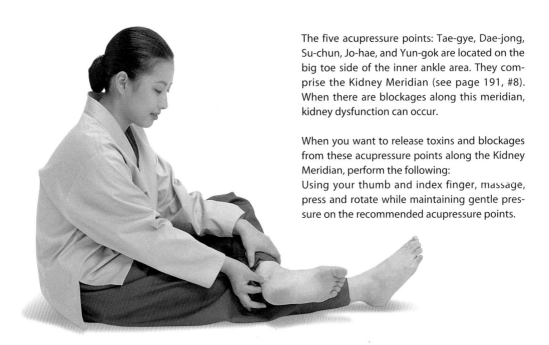

The five acupressure points: Tae-gye, Dae-jong, Su-chun, Jo-hae, and Yun-gok are located on the big toe side of the inner ankle area. They comprise the Kidney Meridian (see page 191, #8). When there are blockages along this meridian, kidney dysfunction can occur.

When you want to release toxins and blockages from these acupressure points along the Kidney Meridian, perform the following:
Using your thumb and index finger, massage, press and rotate while maintaining gentle pressure on the recommended acupressure points.

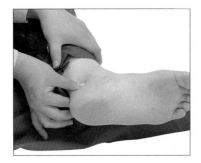

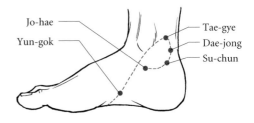

Jo-hae
Yun-gok
Tae-gye
Dae-jong
Su-chun

6. MYUNG-MOON BREATHING TO ACTIVATE KIDNEY FUNCTION

Benefits Myung-moon means the gate of life. Myung-moon point is located opposite of the naval in the spine and this point and the kidneys are located in close proximity to one another. Therefore, Myung-moon breathing enables accumulation of heat energy at the site of the Dahn-jon and kidneys. Water energy activates the kidneys. Ki energy accumulates in the Dahn-jon, warming the kidneys and activating kidney functioning.

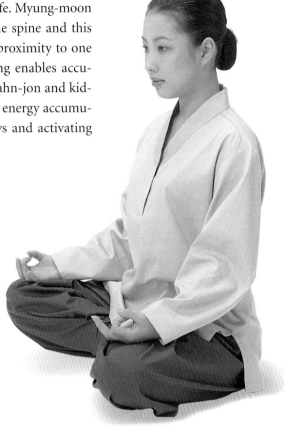

Sit in a half-lotus postion with your hands resting comfortably on the top of your legs, palms facing up. When you inhale, focus on the Myung-moon point becoming warmer. Notice the gentle expansion of the abdomen. When you exhale, slowly pull the abdomen inward. Again, inhale and push the abdomen gently out and down at a 45-degree angle. As you inhale, follow the flow of Ki energy through the Myung-moon and downward towards the Dahn-jon.

Visualize the Myung-moon as the opening in the body and the abdomen as a balloon collecting the Ki. This will foster accumulation of Ki energy in the Dahn-jon. As the kidneys and the Dahn-jon become warmer and warmer, Water energy is activated to enhance the functioning of the kidneys.

Myung-moon

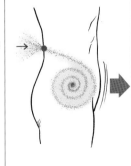

When you inhale, the abdomen expands.

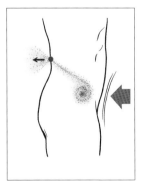

When you exhale, the abdomen contracts.

2) BLADDER INFECTION

Bladder infections occur when there is a proliferation of a virus or bacterium within the bladder membranes, which segue through the urethra to the urinary tract. The infection can re-occur and become chronic. Women tend to have a higher proclivity towards contracting urinary tract infections (URI's) due to the urethra measuring only about 1.5 inches long, thereby facilitating entrance of organisms causing bladder maladies. People who sit for long periods of time are more susceptible to infection because of compression of the bladder. Urinating is the most important artillery in combating and preventing URI's. Drinking water is helpful in the flushing of the troublesome organisms from the body. It is helpful to be mindful of urination and not to prohibit it for many hours at a time, or you can create a breeding ground for infection. For men, it could be the swelling of the prostate gland.

Dahn-jon breathing assists in the accumulation of Ki energy in the Dahn-jon, thereby boosting the immune system and expediting recovery from microbes infesting the bladder. It is recommended that you urinate prior to and following the exercises depicted in this section. Attend to the depth and intensity in the performance of the Dahn-jon breathing accompanying the exercises. This will enable you to derive significant benefit.

SWEEPING DOWN THE BLADDER MERIDIAN (Book 1, p. 99)

Benefits Helps chronic lumbago, waist and lower extremities; promotes a feeling of vitality.

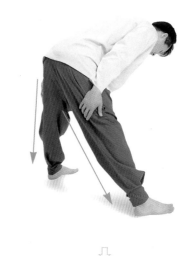

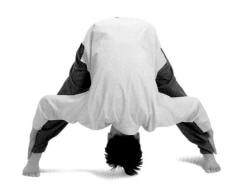

1. LEG SWINGS

TIPS   Do not lock your knee. Keep your knee soft while straightening your leg and utilizing a swinging motion. The waist moves naturally in the opposite direction of the swing.

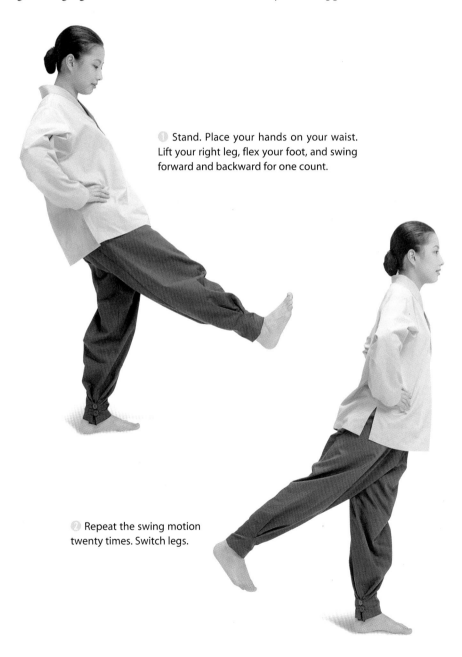

① Stand. Place your hands on your waist. Lift your right leg, flex your foot, and swing forward and backward for one count.

② Repeat the swing motion twenty times. Switch legs.

2. HEEL DROP EXERCISE

TIPS Focus on landing on your heels with the weight of your whole body.

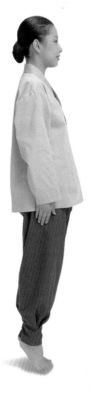

① Stand with your feet together, and your arms at your sides. Inhale. Raise yourself on your toes.

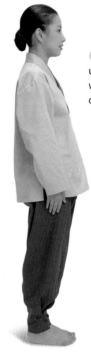

② Exhale. Exaggerate, using a gentle pressure with your whole body, to drop on your heels.

3. RAISED REG FOOT TAPPING

① Lie on your back with your arms extended to the sides. Lift your legs 90-degrees. Maintain soft knees. Flex your feet.

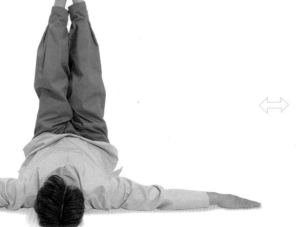

4. FOOT TO FACE LEG STRETCH

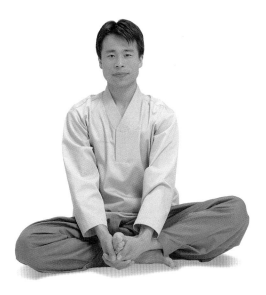

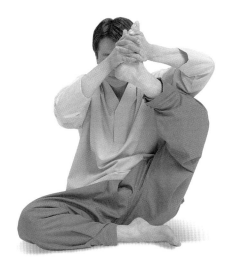

① Sit. Interlock your fingers and cup your left foot.

② Inhale. Gently bring the sole of your foot towards your face. Hold for as long as is comfortable. Exhale and gently lower your foot. Perform the same motions with your right foot. Repeat three times.

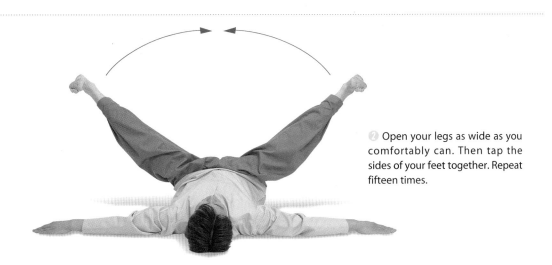

② Open your legs as wide as you comfortably can. Then tap the sides of your feet together. Repeat fifteen times.

3) STAMINA/ STRENGTHENING

When there is a lot of stress and accompanying fatigue in a person's life, there is a decrease in vital energy or stamina. Lack of motivation and sexual desire can occur as well, as can sexual dysfunction, including impotence, or erectile disorder. This can render disruption in intimate partnerships.

It is necessary to strengthen the waist and areas of the body in close proximity to the waist. This can be accomplished by enhancing the kidney energy. Adherents of Eastern Medicine believe that the kidney controls the Jung energy, vital energy in the lower abdomen.

Both the kidney and the liver are vital organs. The kidney is responsible for filtering the blood and the liver detoxifies the body. They must be optimally functioning in order to develop and maintain stamina. If there is weakness in any one of these two organs, sexual functioning can be adversely affected. The Dahnhak Meridian exercises recommended in this chapter will enable optimal kidney and liver functioning and enhance overall vitality for the participant.

BICYCLE EXERCISE
(Book 1, p. 142)

Benefits Strengthens and stimulates lower extremities, muscles and nerves around the perineal region and reproductive glands, thereby enabling heightened stamina.

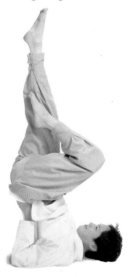

WHEELBARROW POSTURE
(Book 2, p. 87)

TIPS Avoid this exercise if you have hypertension or heart disease.

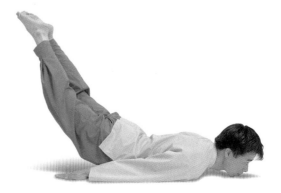

1. HOLDING TORSO LIFT

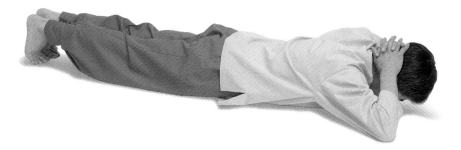

① Lie on your stomach. Flex your toes. Interlock your fingers behind your neck. If the floor is too hard, you can lie on a mat.

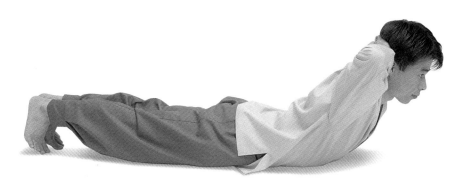

② Slowly and gently lift your trunk for as long as you comfortably can. Gently and slowly lower your trunk to the floor. Repeat ten times.

2. TIP TOE STETCHING

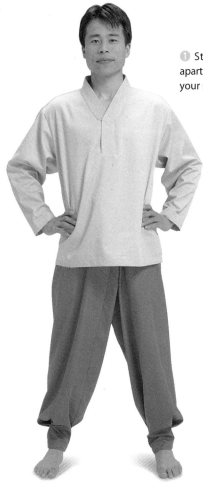

① Stand with your feet shoulder width apart. Place your hands on your waist. Relax your neck and shoulders.

② Inhale. Exhale slowly while bending from your trunk with your palms on the floor and your fingers pointing towards one another.

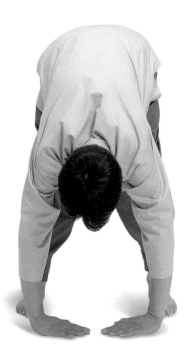

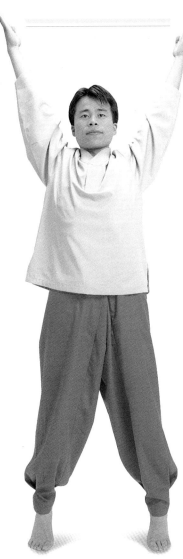

③ Inhale. Raise both of your arms above your head stretching with your palms towards the sky while simultaneously rising on your tip toes. Exhale to the original posture and repeat three times.

ANAL CONTRACTING EXERCISE FOR STAMINA/ STENGTHENING

Benefits Stimulates the Im-maek and Dok-maek. The reproductive system in men will become strengthened with daily practice. Can assist in rectifying sexual dysfunction. For women, this exercise will augment the strengthening of vaginal musculature.

① You can perform this exercise in various positions: Sitting in a half-lotus postion, as well as standing. Concentrate on lengthening the spine while performing this exercise.
② Inhale as you distend your lower abdomen. Hold while contracting your anus.
③ Continue to hold for as long as you are comfortable. Exhale and relax the anus, while contracting the abdominal muscles, bringing them towards your back. Perform this exercise for about five minutes. You can increase the time as you practice with consistency.

3. SIT-UP WITH FORWARD BEND

Benefits Strengthens the kidneys and waist area. Helps correct sexual dysfunction.

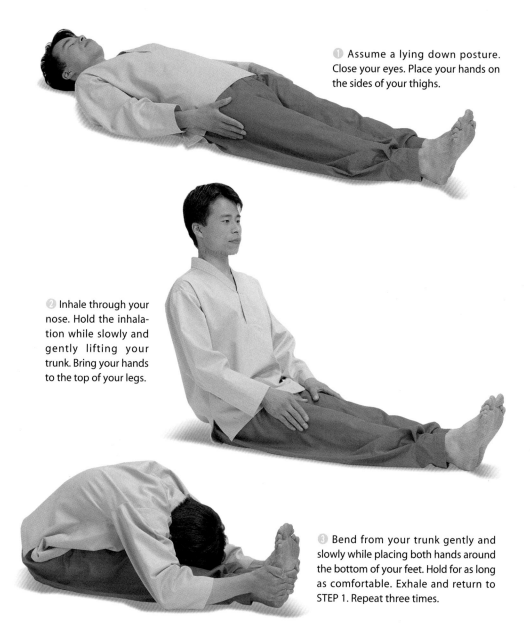

① Assume a lying down posture. Close your eyes. Place your hands on the sides of your thighs.

② Inhale through your nose. Hold the inhalation while slowly and gently lifting your trunk. Bring your hands to the top of your legs.

③ Bend from your trunk gently and slowly while placing both hands around the bottom of your feet. Hold for as long as comfortable. Exhale and return to STEP 1. Repeat three times.

4. THIGH TAPPING AND STRETCHING

Benefits Stimulates and strengthens the autonomic nervous system, particularly the reproductive gland. Strengthens stamina and improves sexual dysfunction.

TIPS It is important to focus on the Dahn-jon and relax the muscles in the thighs and legs as you perform this exercise.

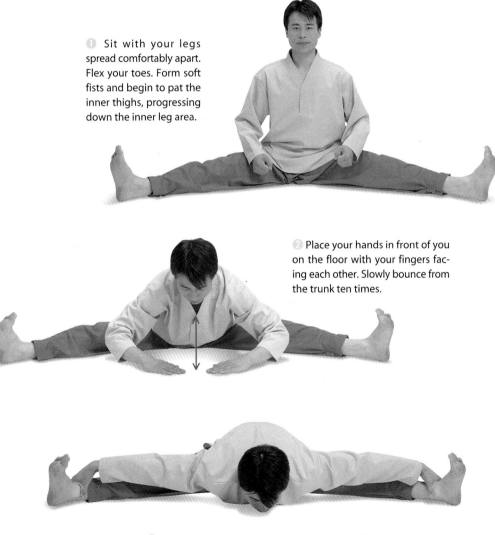

① Sit with your legs spread comfortably apart. Flex your toes. Form soft fists and begin to pat the inner thighs, progressing down the inner leg area.

② Place your hands in front of you on the floor with your fingers facing each other. Slowly bounce from the trunk ten times.

③ Inhale. Bend from the trunk and place both of your hands on your ankles with your chin reaching towards the floor. Repeat three times.

5. TWISTING SIDE TO SIDE WITH LEGS RAISED

Benefits Strengthens abdominal muscles to increase stamina and optimal sexual functioning. Prevents and helps reduce symptoms of lumbago. Prevents urological and reproductive related disorders.

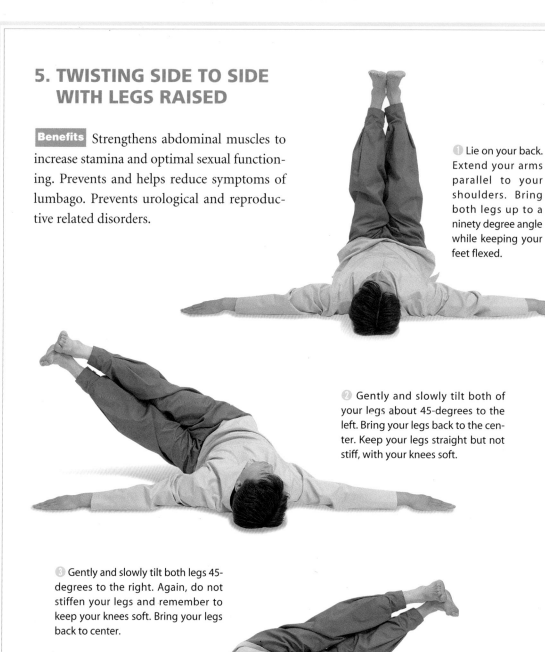

① Lie on your back. Extend your arms parallel to your shoulders. Bring both legs up to a ninety degree angle while keeping your feet flexed.

② Gently and slowly tilt both of your legs about 45-degrees to the left. Bring your legs back to the center. Keep your legs straight but not stiff, with your knees soft.

③ Gently and slowly tilt both legs 45-degrees to the right. Again, do not stiffen your legs and remember to keep your knees soft. Bring your legs back to center.

④ Repeat ten times.

6. RAISING HEELS AND BALANCING

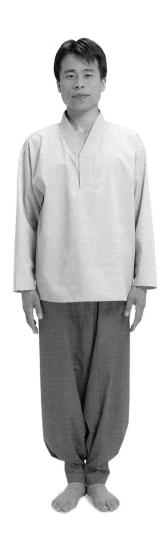

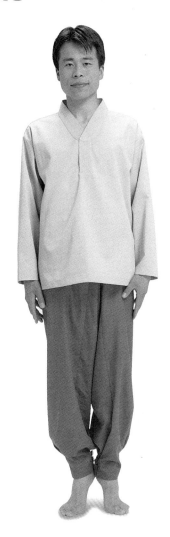

① Stand. Place your heels together with your toes apart, about three inches. Place hands at your sides.

② Inhale. Lift your heels as much as you can. Keep your heels together as you perform this motion. Hold your breath while simultaneously tightening the anal sphincter and the hip and leg muscles, and imagine pulling them towards your perineum. Focus on the perineal area.

③ Exhale. Relax. Slowly lower your heels. Repeat ten times.

1) EXERCISES FOR PREGNANCY

❁

The process of birthing necessitates a tremendous surge of energy within a short period of time. In preparation for the labor, it is beneficial during the pregnancy to perform the recommended Dahnhak Meridian exercises to accumulate the vital Ki energy necessary to build, condition and maintain a healthy body, mind and spirit, and assist in the challenge of labor. This can help to mitigate unnecessary suffering that can occur in the labor itself as well as in later years.

The Meridian exercises recommended in this chapter are different from other exercises, as consideration for the growing fetus is highlighted and accounted for. Specific precautions include: breathing naturally, as opposed to holding inhalations, or intensifying breathing patterns. When assuming a Hang-gong posture, do not raise your legs; rather keep them on the floor. Close your eyes and progress in your relaxation as you concentrate and converse with your growing fetus.

FIRST TRIMESTER (0-4 MONTHS)

This period of time requires an attempt on your part to be in touch with your body's natural rhythms, instead of forcing yourself to become unnecessarily distressed. Relaxing is extremely important for you and your developing baby.

TWISTING KNEES TO TOUCH THE FLOOR (Book 2, p. 56)

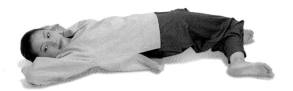

1. ANKLE JOINT EXERCISE

Benefits When you rotate your ankles, it opens up blockages to allow Ki energy and blood circulation to the lower extremities. Assists optimal reproductive system functioning and pregnancy.

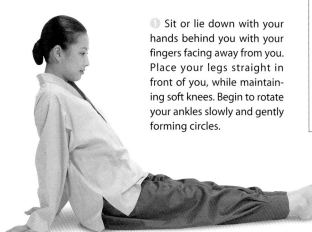

① Sit or lie down with your hands behind you with your fingers facing away from you. Place your legs straight in front of you, while maintaining soft knees. Begin to rotate your ankles slowly and gently forming circles.

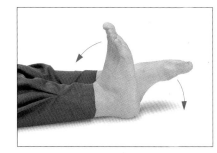

② Slowly alternate flexing and extending your feet. Focus on the muscles tightening and releasing.

2. WHOLE BODY STRETCH

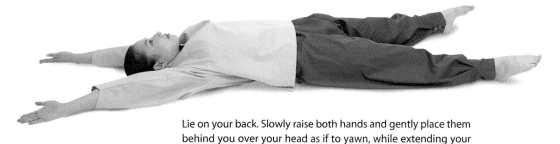

Lie on your back. Slowly raise both hands and gently place them behind you over your head as if to yawn, while extending your feet. You can also perform this by locking your fingers.

3. PUSH-UP WITH KNEE SUPPORT

Benefits This posture is specifically modified for the pregnant woman, as it reduces excess pressure in the abdominal area.

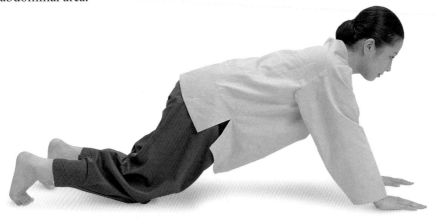

① Bend your knees. Flex your toes and place your hands in front of you, with your fingers facing away from you.

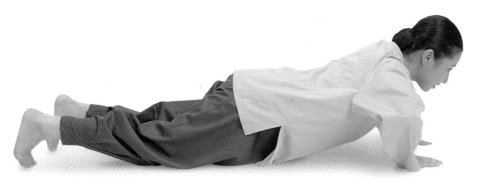

② Gently expand your chest, bend your elbows and lower your upper body. Begin by performing five times. Increase as you progress in this practice.

4. HIP LIFT

Benefits Strengthens and improves the elasticity of the pelvis. Digestion and elimination is enhanced.

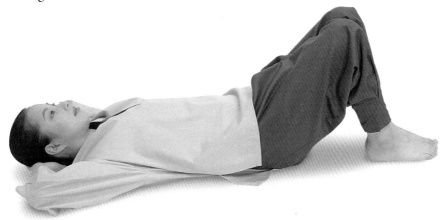

① Lie on your back with your knees bent. Lock your fingers behind your neck. Open your legs while bringing your heels close to your hips.

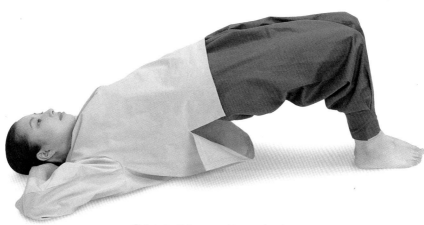

② Inhale. Raise your hips and waist. Touch knees together while contracting your pelvis.

③ Exhale. Lower your hips and waist. Repeat three times.

5. SIDE LEG LIFT

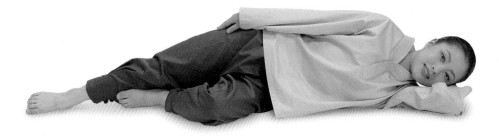

① Lie on your left side. Form
a pillow with your left arm
and rest head comfortably.

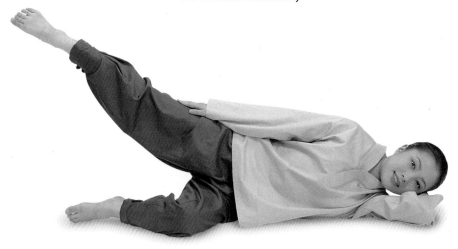

② Bend your left knee. Place your right
hand on your right thigh. Inhale. Raise
your right leg up. Exhale and bring it
down. Repeat ten to twenty times. Turn
on your right side and repeat leg lifting with your left leg.

6. CIRCULATION EXERCISE

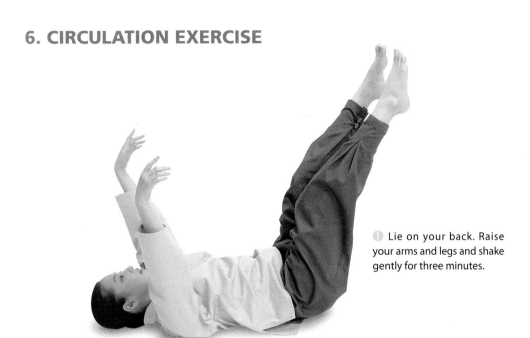

① Lie on your back. Raise your arms and legs and shake gently for three minutes.

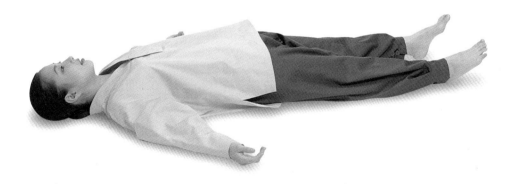

② Drop your arms and legs. Relax your body.

During this period of time, the fetus is settled in the uterus, thereby decreasing the liability to the mother and fetus. Exercise levels can be increased with more comfort and safety, though with caution and with the approval of your labor and delivery consultant. Appetite is usually enhanced during this time and the nourishment will provide the energy necessary to perform the following exercises. The Meridian exercises recommended in this section will facilitate the conditioning of the body to be strong in preparation for the ensuing months of pregnancy, including labor and delivery.

1. SHOULDER SHRUGGING

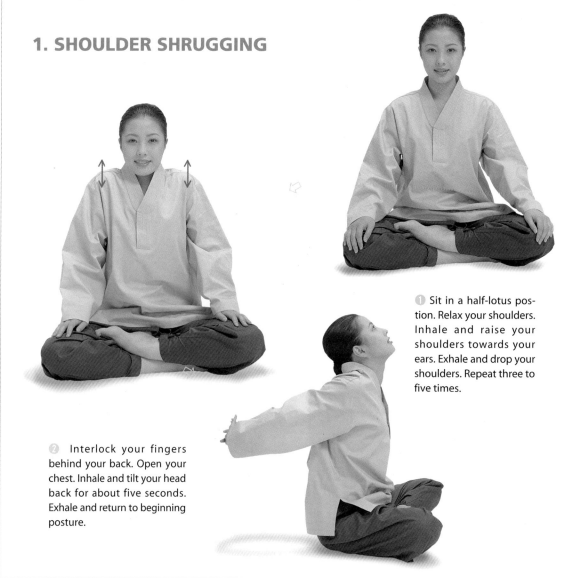

❶ Sit in a half-lotus position. Relax your shoulders. Inhale and raise your shoulders towards your ears. Exhale and drop your shoulders. Repeat three to five times.

❷ Interlock your fingers behind your back. Open your chest. Inhale and tilt your head back for about five seconds. Exhale and return to beginning posture.

2. SITTING SIDE BEND WITH ARM STETCH

Benefits Promotes elasticity, flexibility and mobility to the waist and sides of trunk area while preventing and lessening discomfort.

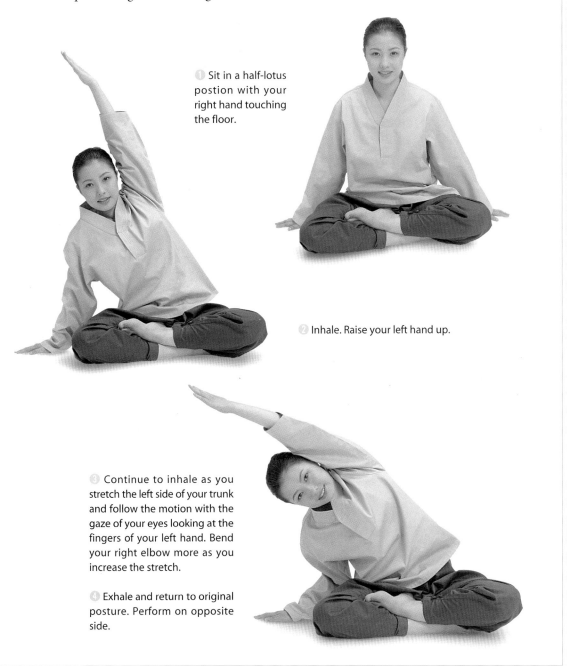

① Sit in a half-lotus postion with your right hand touching the floor.

② Inhale. Raise your left hand up.

③ Continue to inhale as you stretch the left side of your trunk and follow the motion with the gaze of your eyes looking at the fingers of your left hand. Bend your right elbow more as you increase the stretch.

④ Exhale and return to original posture. Perform on opposite side.

3. BUTTERFLY FLAPPING

TIPS   Jang-gang acupressure point is located in the region of the coccyx and perineum. When you stimulate the Jang-gang point and perineal area, perform this naturally without force. This exercise stimulates the Jang-gang point. When you perform this exercise flap your legs gently without causing strain. It is recommended that you sit on a blanket or mat to provide more cushioning for you and your fetus.

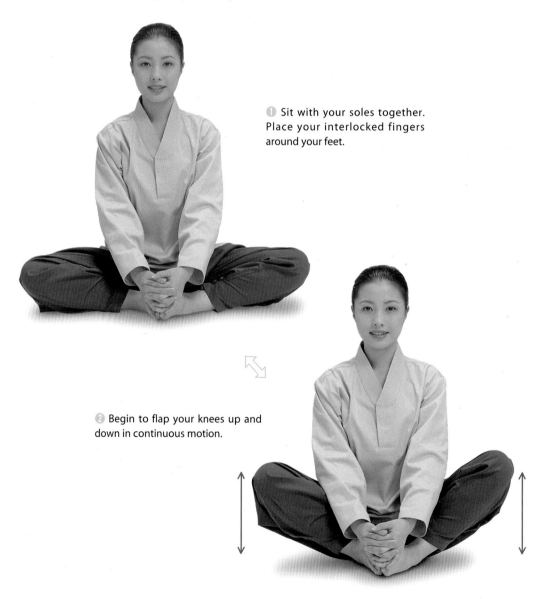

❶ Sit with your soles together. Place your interlocked fingers around your feet.

❷ Begin to flap your knees up and down in continuous motion.

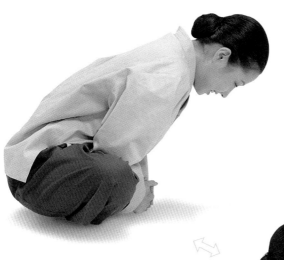

③ Lean forward with your upper body and rock back and forth, while lifting your hips up and down to stimulate the Jang-gang point and perineum.

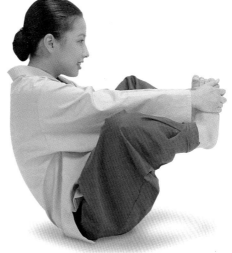

④ While continuing to grasp your feet with your hands, slightly tilt your upper body backwards to keep your balance. Hold for as long as you comfortably can. This will stimulate the Jang-gang point and perineal area.

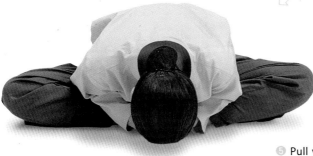

⑤ Pull your feet towards your body while gently and slowly lowering your upper trunk and your head towards your feet as much as you can without straining.

4. CAT STRETCH

Benefits Beneficial for pregnancy. Helps placement of uterus to accommodate increasing size and necessary mobility for the developing fetus.

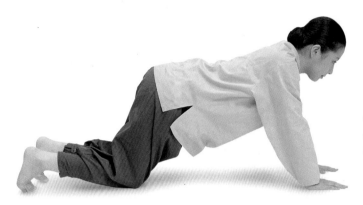

① Assume posture on hands and knees with your toes pointing towards your body.

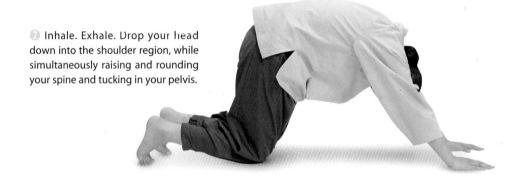

② Inhale. Exhale. Drop your head down into the shoulder region, while simultaneously raising and rounding your spine and tucking in your pelvis.

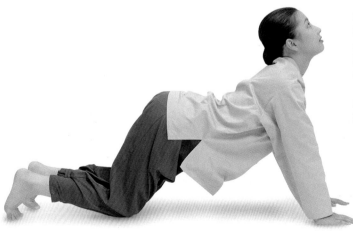

③ Inhale. Exhale and raise your head and look towards the horizon and sky. Simultaneously lower and arch your spine downward into a Lion Posture.

④ Inhale. Return to Step 1. Repeat three to five times.

5. SITTING SIDE BEND VARIATION

Benefits Realigns the pelvis. Enhances Ki energy and blood circulation as it warms the lower abdomen.

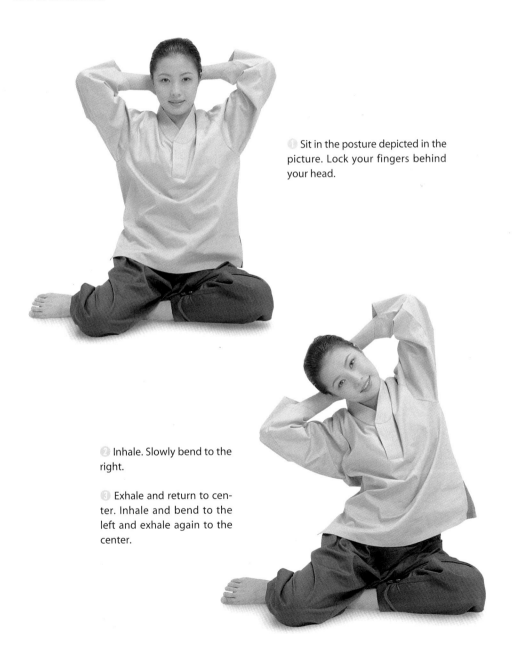

① Sit in the posture depicted in the picture. Lock your fingers behind your head.

② Inhale. Slowly bend to the right.

③ Exhale and return to center. Inhale and bend to the left and exhale again to the center.

During this trimester, anxiety can mount as the pregnant woman anticipates the birth of the baby. It is helpful to apply measures that will boost the mind/body/spirit towards optimal relaxation. Listening to peaceful music along with other things that you associate with a relaxed state of mind is helpful. Following the recommended exercises in this section along with Dahn-jon breathing will be significantly helpful towards this goal.

1. SQUATS WITH TURNED OUT FEET

Benefits Strengthens thigh muscles and external genital region, and anal sphincter muscle. Facilitates release of muscular tension to ease the passage through the birth canal and decrease pain. With the increased weight gain during this trimester, the woman can become more sedentary and fatigued, and may therefore be tempted to exercise less, thereby experiencing muscular weakness. The increase in the strength of the thigh muscle will assist in the opening of the pelvis to help push the baby through the birth canal with more feasibility.

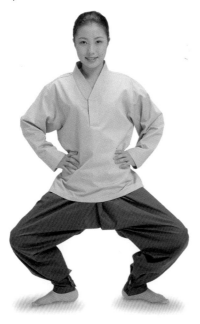

❶ Stand with your hands on your waist with your toes pointing outwards and your heels facing one another.

❷ Inhale. Bend your knees. Exhale, and stand up. Repeat twelve times.

2. KNEELING AND ARCHING

Benefits Strengthens and realigns the spine, waist and legs to decrease pain during delivery.

TIPS If surface is too hard for the knee, perform on a mat.

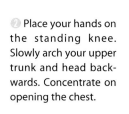

❷ Place your hands on the standing knee. Slowly arch your upper trunk and head backwards. Concentrate on opening the chest.

❶ Kneel on one knee, with your toes facing your body. Bend and stand on your other knee with your thigh parallel to the ground as shown in the picture.

STRADDLE STRETCH (Book 2, p. 134)

TIPS Bend slowly and gently so as not to create undue pressure on your abdomen.

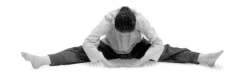

3. LEG LIFT

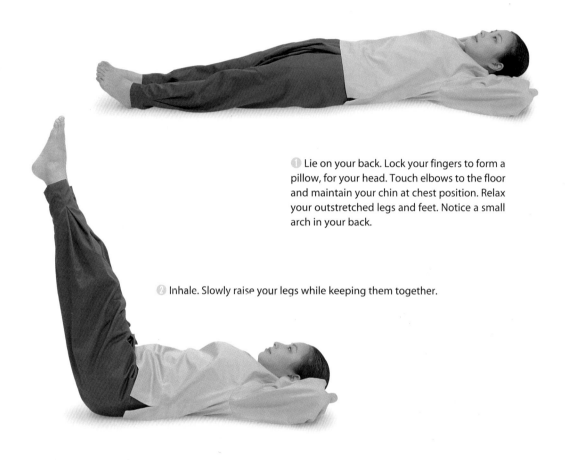

① Lie on your back. Lock your fingers to form a pillow, for your head. Touch elbows to the floor and maintain your chin at chest position. Relax your outstretched legs and feet. Notice a small arch in your back.

② Inhale. Slowly raise your legs while keeping them together.

③ Exhale. Slowly lower your legs but do not touch the floor. Repeat STEPs 2 and 3 five times.

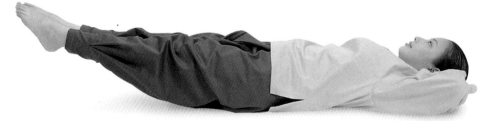

4. WAIST LIFT

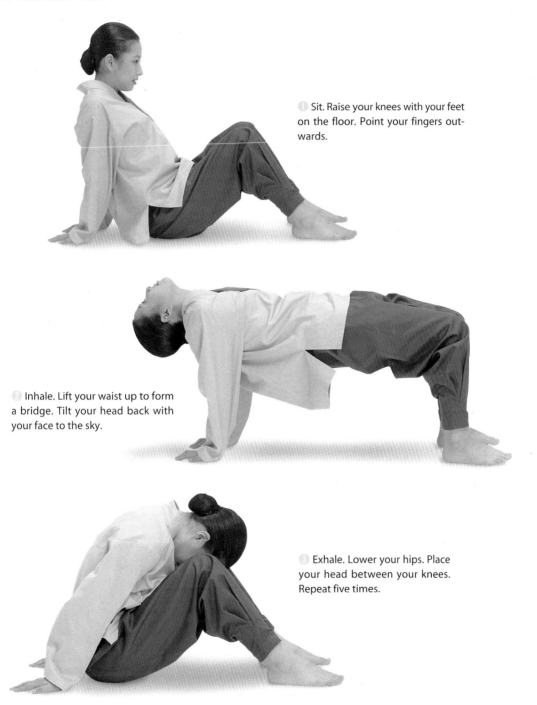

① Sit. Raise your knees with your feet on the floor. Point your fingers outwards.

② Inhale. Lift your waist up to form a bridge. Tilt your head back with your face to the sky.

③ Exhale. Lower your hips. Place your head between your knees. Repeat five times.

5. BABY POSTURE

TIPS Breathe naturally without forcefully pushing your abdomen in and out.

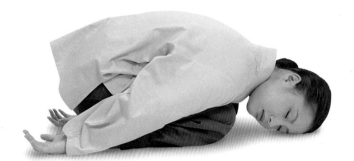

Assume posture depicted in the picture. Place your knees apart. Your head can face in either direction. Drop your arms comfortably with your palms facing up.

6. RESTING WITH FEET ELEVATED AGAINST THE WALL

Benefits This posture is very important for relieving fatigue for the pregnant woman as well as for people who stand on their feet a lot.

Lie down with your arms stretched out to your sides at shoulder level. Bring your hips close to the wall. Raise your legs with your feet shoulder width apart. Breathe normally and comfortably.

7. TIGHTING FISTS AND STRETCHING WITH PRAYER HANDS

TIPS   When first performing this exercise repeat slowly ten times. As you progress in your practice, you can increase to thirty times at a faster pace

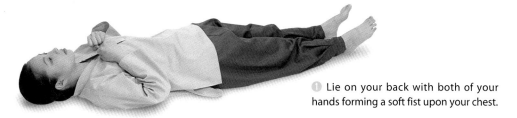

① Lie on your back with both of your hands forming a soft fist upon your chest.

② Form a strong fist. Open and close very forcefully fifteen times.

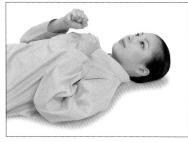

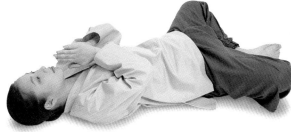

③ Place your hands in prayer posture, while bringing the soles of your feet together.

④ Inhale. Exhale. Place your arms over your head with palms together and feet relaxed.

⑤ Inhale. Return to STEP 3 and repeat.

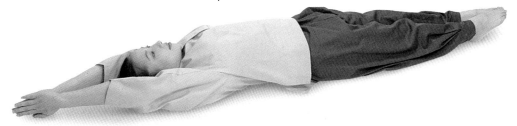

2) RECOVERY FROM POST PARTUM

Immediately following birth, the bones of a woman are soft and the joints and organs need to be realigned. Two or three days of maximum rest are needed to begin the healing process. Minimal activity is recommended to prevent hemorrhaging over the initial six-week post partum time period.

The recommended Meridian exercises in this section are particularly beneficial to the post partum woman. They begin with lying postures and proceed to standing postures. It is important to proceed with caution and be watchful not to strain your joints and muscles during your exercise movements. Practice these exercises for about a two-month time period and consult with your labor and delivery consultant before proceeding to the standing postures.

ANKLE JOINT EXERCISE
(Book 2, p. 103)

Benefits Stimulates bladder meridian and strengthens reproductive system. Enhances function of the stomach and liver.

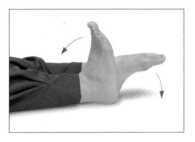

TIGHTENING FISTS (Book 2, p. 119)

Benefits Helps blood circulation and decreases swelling in arms and hands.

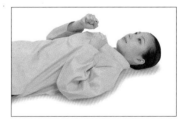

1. WAIST MOVEMENT EXERCISE

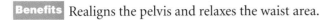 **Benefits** Realigns the pelvis and relaxes the waist area.

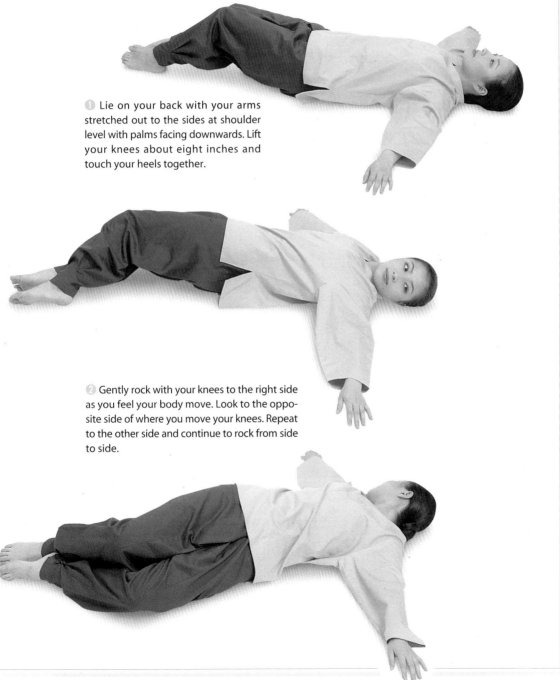

① Lie on your back with your arms stretched out to the sides at shoulder level with palms facing downwards. Lift your knees about eight inches and touch your heels together.

② Gently rock with your knees to the right side as you feel your body move. Look to the opposite side of where you move your knees. Repeat to the other side and continue to rock from side to side.

2. PELVIS EXERCISE

TIPS Perform each motion very slowly.

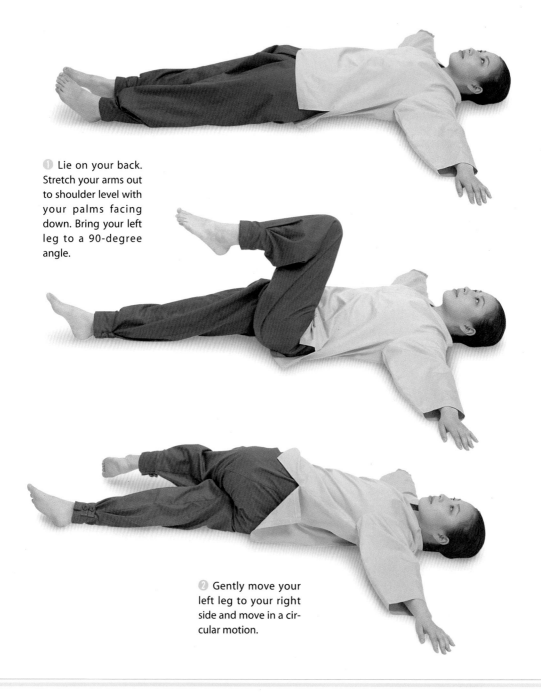

① Lie on your back. Stretch your arms out to shoulder level with your palms facing down. Bring your left leg to a 90-degree angle.

② Gently move your left leg to your right side and move in a circular motion.

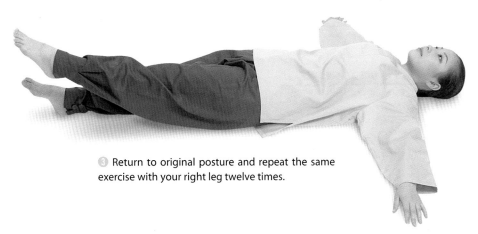

③ Return to original posture and repeat the same exercise with your right leg twelve times.

3. DAHN-JON BREATHING

Benefits At the time of the birth, the mother and baby expend Ki energy, thereby rendering a deficit in the mother's overall Ki energy supply. In order to replenish, accumulate, and re-vitalize the harmonious symmetry and realignment of the body, Dahn-jon breathing is essential.

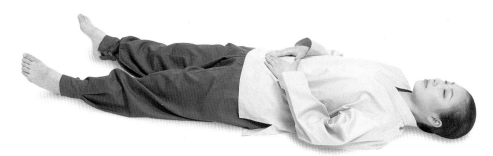

① Lie on your back. Form a triangle with your hands and place them on your Dahn-jon. Focus on your lower abdomen.

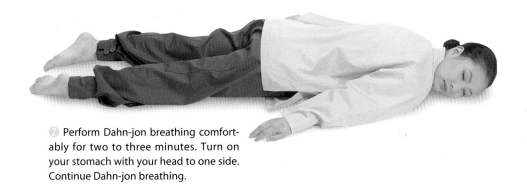

② Perform Dahn-jon breathing comfortably for two to three minutes. Turn on your stomach with your head to one side. Continue Dahn-jon breathing.

3) LEUKORRHEA

Leukorrhea, or discharge from the vagina, is experienced by many women. It is accompanied by a sensation of a chill around the waist, lower abdomen and the knees, even though the air is a warm temperature. It can, if untreated cause irregular menstruation and infertility problems. It results from the malfunction of blood circulation in the lower extremities and the imbalance of the sexual hormones after birth, miscarriage and birth control medicines and appliances. Certain foods can be helpful to increase body warmth, such as ginger root, potatoes, onions and radish. It is best to avoid artificial seasonings as well as to avoid sugar.

The recommended exercises in this section will concentrate on assisting those with leukorrhea to enhance the depth of Dahn-jon breathing and expel coldness from the body. People with hypertension should avoid breathing with this intensity and proceed to Dahn-jon breathing as regularly prescribed. Within two to three months you should be able to noticeably recognize an increase in your body temperature. Initially, you may experience a worsening of your symptoms, i.e., sensation of chills, body aches, etc. However, with consistent practice, you will notice a diminishing of symptoms related to leukorrhea, and an overall, positive change in your sense of well-being.

BODY TAPPING
(Book 1, p. 22)

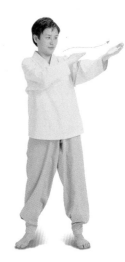

CIRCULATION EXERCISE
(Book 1, p. 26)

Benefits Helps blood circulation and decreases edema in hands and arms

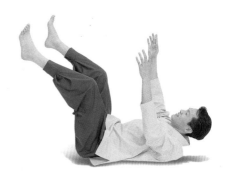

SITTING FORWARD BEND
(Book 1, p. 52)

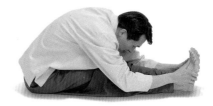

BRIDGE POSTURE
(Book 2, p. 58)

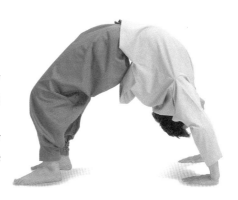

Benefits Flexes whole body particularly the neck, hips, waist and shoulders; releases tension.

Controls Yin-Yang Ki energy flow thereby harmonizing the balance in the body.

1. TAILBONE TAPPING

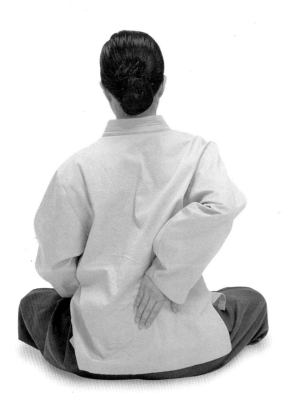

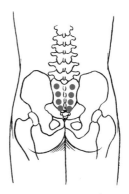

Eight acupressure points around tailbone

Around the tailbone, there are eight acupressure points. When there is a blockage in the points, the intestines harden and Ki energy cannot freely flow. There is increased coldness and leukorrhea can result. The sexual organs can be affected as well. From a sitting position, place the palm of your hand gently on the tailbone area. Gently pat the areas where the acupressure points are located.

2. PALM PUSHING WITH BODY TWISTING

TIPS When you perform these movements, focus on keeping your chest open and elongate the spine.

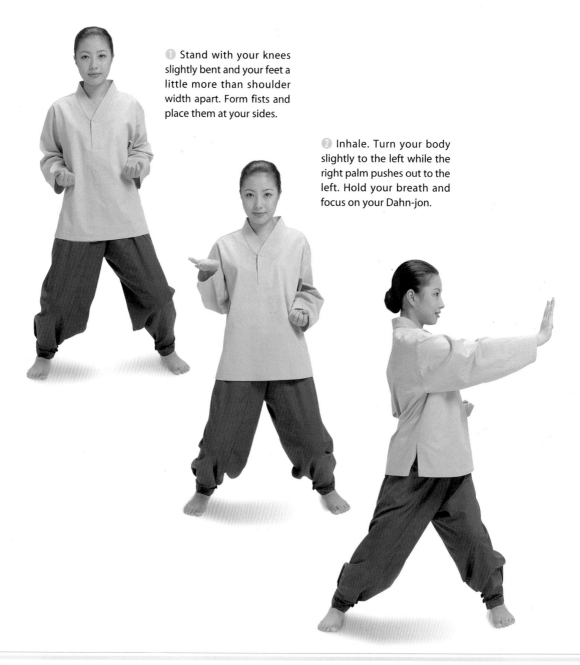

❶ Stand with your knees slightly bent and your feet a little more than shoulder width apart. Form fists and place them at your sides.

❷ Inhale. Turn your body slightly to the left while the right palm pushes out to the left. Hold your breath and focus on your Dahn-jon.

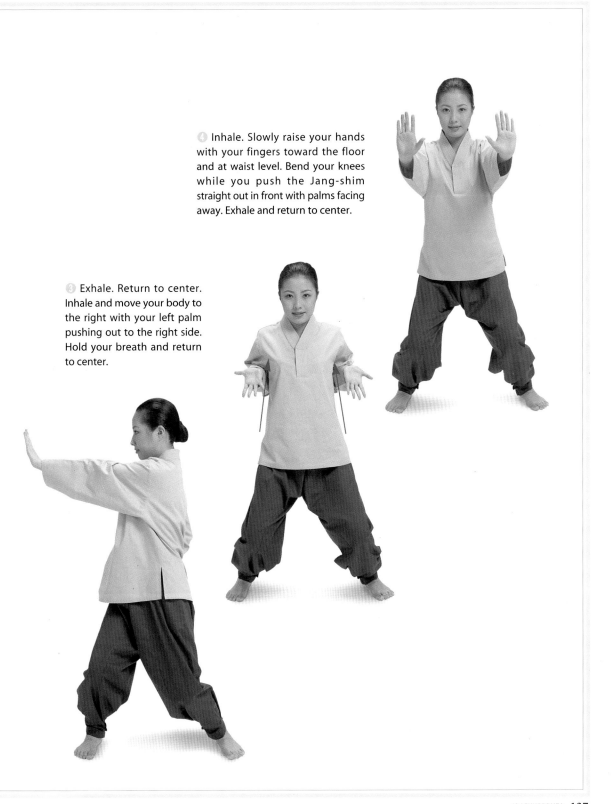

④ Inhale. Slowly raise your hands with your fingers toward the floor and at waist level. Bend your knees while you push the Jang-shim straight out in front with palms facing away. Exhale and return to center.

③ Exhale. Return to center. Inhale and move your body to the right with your left palm pushing out to the right side. Hold your breath and return to center.

3. CROSSED ANKLE BOW POSTURE

Benefits Releases stagnant blood and Ki energy from abdominal area; strengthens spine. Helps leukorrhea and constipation.

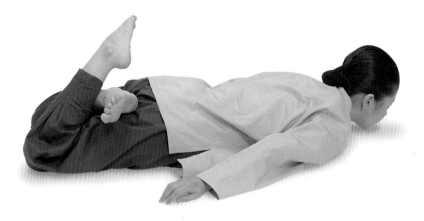

① Lie on your stomach. Bend your knees and cross your feet.

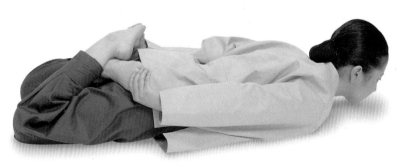

② Hold your feet with both of your hands.

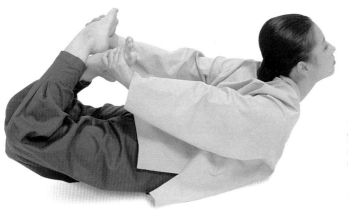

③ Gently pull your feet and gently lift your upper torso and head to form an arch in your back. Hold this position for thirty seconds.

④ Switch feet. Repeat four times.

4. WIGGLING TOES WITH RAISED LEGS

Benefits Helps insomnia, anxiety, headache, low stamina and the cold sensation associated with leukorrhea. The feet house many meridians which are connected to the functioning of the body. Wiggling initiates healing to the body.

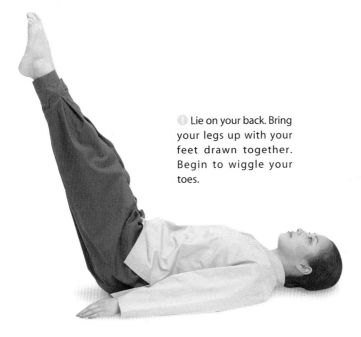

① Lie on your back. Bring your legs up with your feet drawn together. Begin to wiggle your toes.

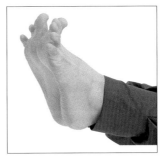

② Rub your toes and feet together. Practice spreading your toes apart as much as possible without touching them with your hands.

5. LEG LIFT VARIATION

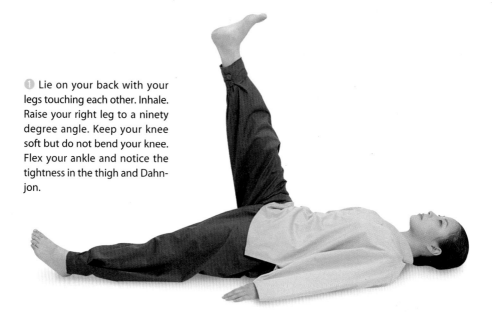

① Lie on your back with your legs touching each other. Inhale. Raise your right leg to a ninety degree angle. Keep your knee soft but do not bend your knee. Flex your ankle and notice the tightness in the thigh and Dahn-jon.

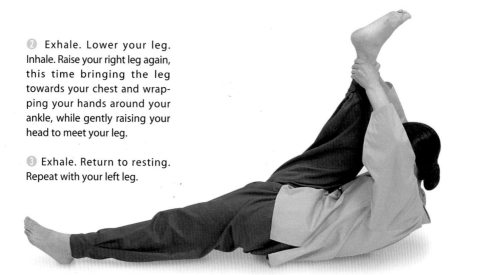

② Exhale. Lower your leg. Inhale. Raise your right leg again, this time bringing the leg towards your chest and wrapping your hands around your ankle, while gently raising your head to meet your leg.

③ Exhale. Return to resting. Repeat with your left leg.

6. KNEELING BACK BEND

TIPS Do not overdo this exercise if you have back pain. Do not perform this exercise if you have hypertension.

① Kneel with your toes flexed under you. Your heels should touch your buttocks.

② Grasp your ankles with your hands. Inhale and raise your Dahn-jon. Simultaneously contract your anus and open your chest.

③ Return to original posture as you exhale.

④ Inhale. Repeat STEP 2.

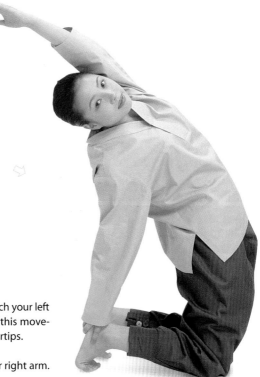

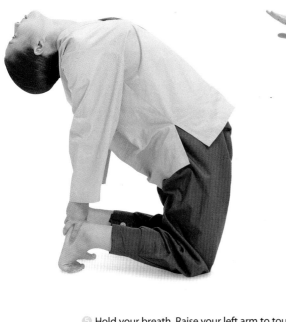

⑤ Hold your breath. Raise your left arm to touch your left ear. Tilt your upper body to the right. Follow this movement with your eyes to gaze at your left fingertips.

⑥ Switch arms and perform STEP 5 with your right arm.

4) MENSTRUAL DISORDERS

Adherents of Eastern Medicine believe that the cramps accompanying menstruation are the result of coldness and stagnant blood, particularly in the area of the pelvis. When there is a blockage or stagnant blood surrounding the pelvis, uterus, and ovaries, weakened functioning of these areas can occur. Some of the symptoms may include fatigue, headache, anxiety, hypersensitivity, and cramps in the abdomen. When the pain is severe, women can experience spasms caused by twisting of the intestines. Excessive bleeding can occur here. Menstrual cramping can occur if there is blockage in the Im-maek, low Ki energy in the kidney, and overall body fragility.

The recommended Meridian exercises will benefit women who suffer from the discomfort of menstrual pain, irregular menstruation, and diseases that affect the uterus. In addition to performing the recommended exercises, it can be helpful to lie on your stomach on a warm surface (or on a heating pad). This will facilitate a sense of serenity and a dissipation of the cramping. Also, rub your hands and place them on your abdomen, rubbing clockwise to help attenuate pain. And lastly, avoid excessive Meridian exercises during menstruation time.

LYING HIP BOUNCE (Book 1, p. 100)

Benefits Opens the Myung-moon acupressure point. Enhances functioning of essential organs and helps lower back pain.

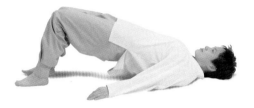

FORWARD BEND FOR WAIST AND HIPS (Book 1, p. 125)

Benefits Helps circulate Ki energy to lower abdomen to release menstrual cramping and irregular menstruation. Calms the mind and enhances radiance of the skin.

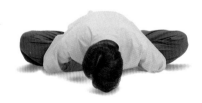

WHEELBARROW POSTURE (Book 2, p. 86)

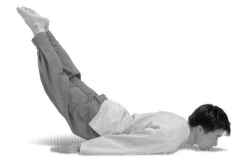

1. PRESSING THE SAM-EUM-GYO ACUPRESSURE POINTS

Benefits Helps relieve knee pain, uterine bleeding, and excessive bleeding during menstruation; helps reproductive problems in women and men.

TIPS Do not press too hard on the Sam-eum-gyo points if you are pregnant.

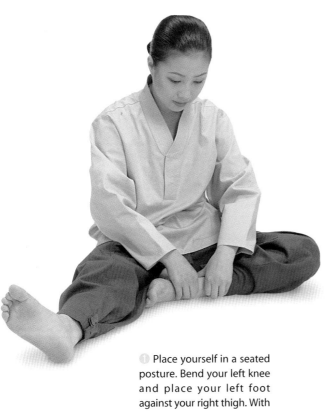

Sam-eum-gyo : located about three fingers width from the inner ankle.

① Place yourself in a seated posture. Bend your left knee and place your left foot against your right thigh. With both thumbs, press on your Sam-eum-gyo point.

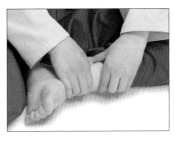

② Inhale. Press your Sam-eum-gyo. Hold your breath and focus on your thumbs. Apply upper body weight as you press on this acupressure point.

③ Exhale. Release your thumbs.

2. STRADDLE STRETCH

Benefits This exercise is particularly beneficial for conditions of diabetes and menstrual cramping. It assists in eliminating fats from the thighs and the abdominal area. Helpful in realigning the lumbar and sacral area of the spine.

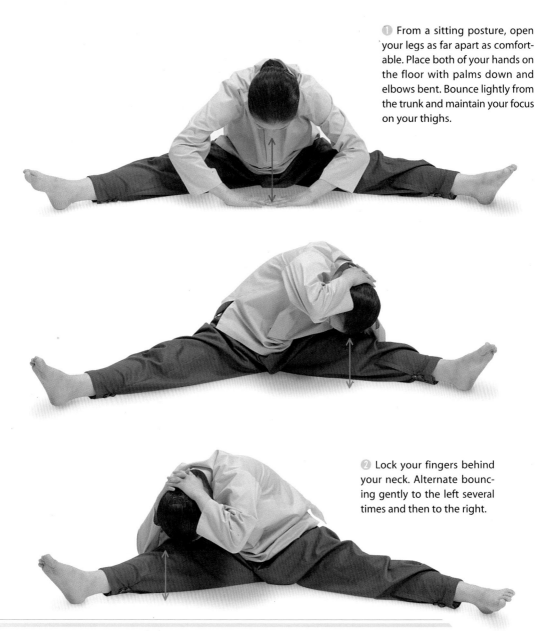

❶ From a sitting posture, open your legs as far apart as comfortable. Place both of your hands on the floor with palms down and elbows bent. Bounce lightly from the trunk and maintain your focus on your thighs.

❷ Lock your fingers behind your neck. Alternate bouncing gently to the left several times and then to the right.

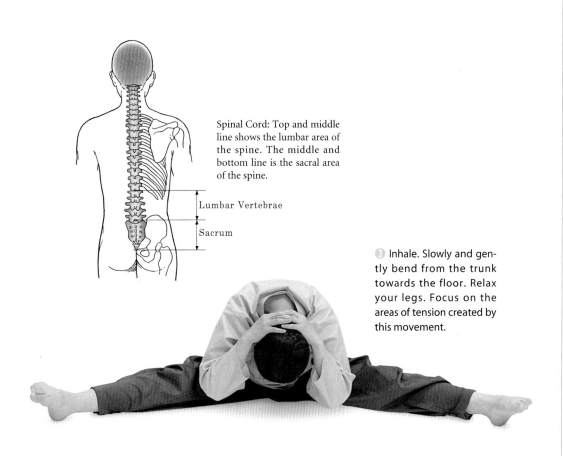

Spinal Cord: Top and middle line shows the lumbar area of the spine. The middle and bottom line is the sacral area of the spine.

Lumbar Vertebrae

Sacrum

③ Inhale. Slowly and gently bend from the trunk towards the floor. Relax your legs. Focus on the areas of tension created by this movement.

PRESSING THE SHIN-YU AND THE JI-SHIL ACUPRESSURE POINTS (Book 2, p. 84)

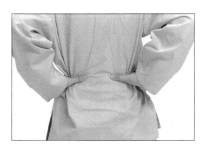

Benefits When you press the Shim-yu and the Ji-Shil acupressure points, it helps to relieve lumbago pain. It helps kidney function and reproductive disorders in men and women.

3. BENDING WITH PRAYER HANDS

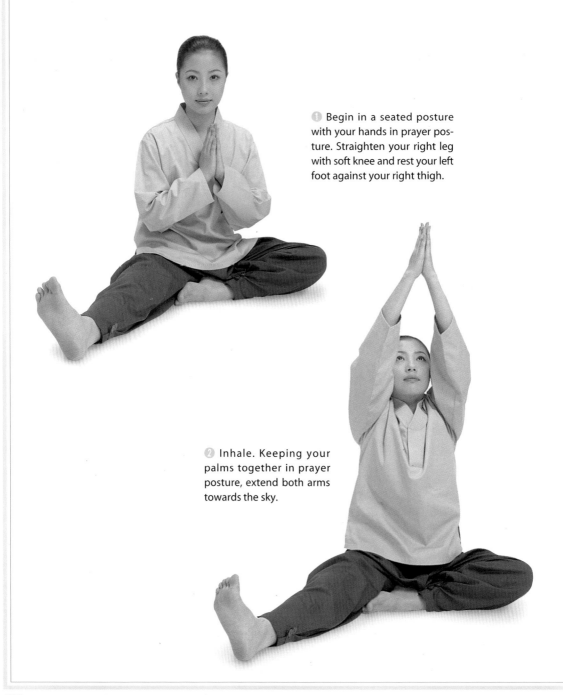

❶ Begin in a seated posture with your hands in prayer posture. Straighten your right leg with soft knee and rest your left foot against your right thigh.

❷ Inhale. Keeping your palms together in prayer posture, extend both arms towards the sky.

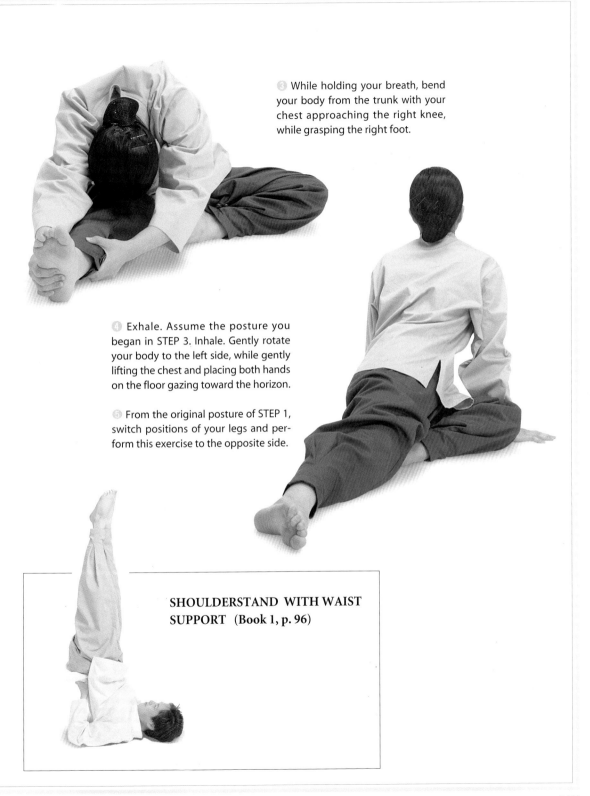

③ While holding your breath, bend your body from the trunk with your chest approaching the right knee, while grasping the right foot.

④ Exhale. Assume the posture you began in STEP 3. Inhale. Gently rotate your body to the left side, while gently lifting the chest and placing both hands on the floor gazing toward the horizon.

⑤ From the original posture of STEP 1, switch positions of your legs and perform this exercise to the opposite side.

SHOULDERSTAND WITH WAIST SUPPORT (Book 1, p. 96)

1) OBESITY

Obesity results from the accumulation of exorbitant amounts of fat(adipose tissue) within the body. It can increase the risk of contracting a multitude of diseases and conditions, including diabetes, stroke, heart disease, certain types of cancer, respiratory functioning, development of gall stones, sleep apnea, high blood pressure and a host of others.

There are three types of muscles: skeletal muscle, smooth muscle and cardiac muscle. The Dahnhak Meridian exercises recommended in this section will facilitate the excretion of the accumulation of excess fats from the body. The function of the intestines will be enhanced by performing these exercises as well, as the blood and Ki energy circulation of the digestive system is stimulated. This will revitalize the brain cells and the metabolic system, igniting fat burning activity, and normalizing hormone secretions. Appetite control and management will become facilitated through continued and consistent practice of these exercises. Through the synthesis of these changes, one can begin to notice a more positive attitude towards life.

BODY TAPPING (Book 1, p. 22)

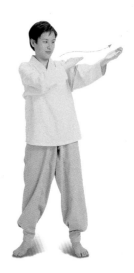

DAHN-JON TAPPING (Book 1, p. 27)

Benefits Relieves gas accumulation from the intestine and eliminates fat from the lower abdomen.

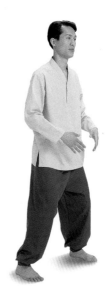

INTESTINE EXERCISE
(Book 1, p. 28)

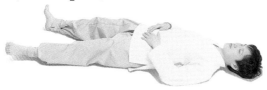

BICYCLE EXERCISE
(Book1, p. 142)

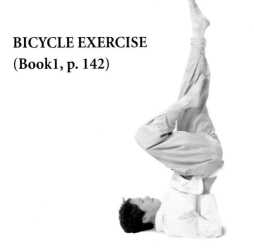

SQUATS WITH TURNED OUT
FEET (Book 2, p. 114)

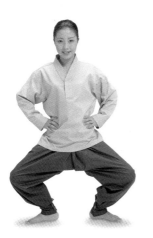

PULLING KNEES TO CHEST
(Book 1, p. 107)

Benefits Realigns pelvis and removes gas from the intestine. Helps to strengthen and lift the buttocks

ARM TWIST (Book 2, p. 14)

Benefits When you perform this exercise, it enhances flexibility in the joints of the wrists, arms, and shoulder blades. Breaks down the fats of the arm muscle to promote leanness. Helps to lessen fatigue and numbness and tingling in the arms.

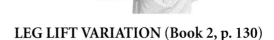

LEG LIFT VARIATION (Book 2, p. 130)

Benefits Relieves accumulation of stagnant blood and toxins from the lower extremities and eliminates fat accumulation from the abdomen and thigh areas.

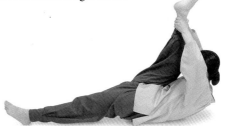

1. SIDE BEND

Benefits Waist, legs and sides become more shapely. Helps to reduce saggy appearance around the shoulders and under arms.

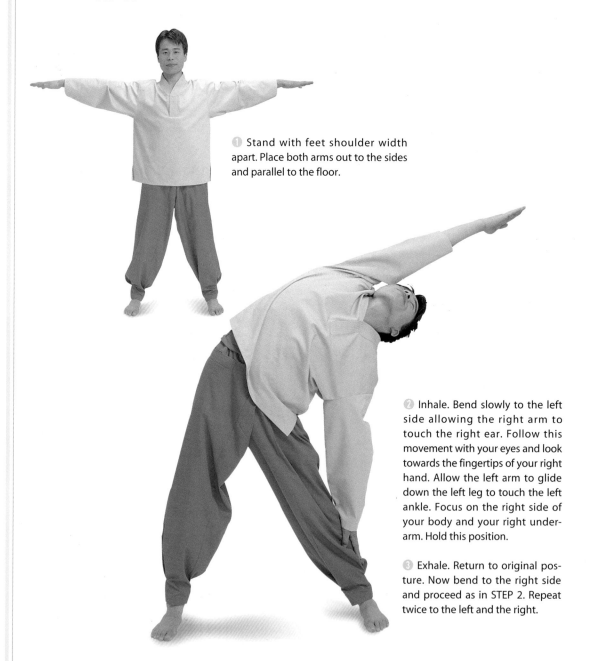

❶ Stand with feet shoulder width apart. Place both arms out to the sides and parallel to the floor.

❷ Inhale. Bend slowly to the left side allowing the right arm to touch the right ear. Follow this movement with your eyes and look towards the fingertips of your right hand. Allow the left arm to glide down the left leg to touch the left ankle. Focus on the right side of your body and your right underarm. Hold this position.

❸ Exhale. Return to original posture. Now bend to the right side and proceed as in STEP 2. Repeat twice to the left and the right.

2. GROIN STRETCH

Benefits Flexes the joint of the leg and the ankle. Strengthens thighs and buttocks. Helps to increase shapeliness of the legs and hips.

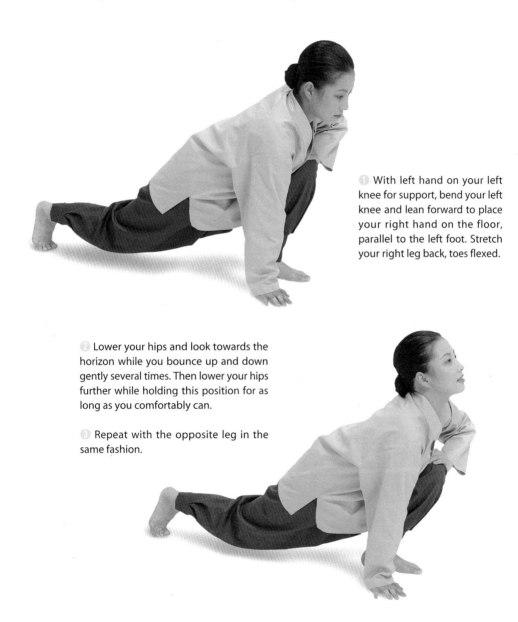

① With left hand on your left knee for support, bend your left knee and lean forward to place your right hand on the floor, parallel to the left foot. Stretch your right leg back, toes flexed.

② Lower your hips and look towards the horizon while you bounce up and down gently several times. Then lower your hips further while holding this position for as long as you comfortably can.

③ Repeat with the opposite leg in the same fashion.

3. GRINDING MOTION WITH LEGS OUTSTRETCHED

Benefits Enhances liver and digestive system function. Flexes waist and legs. Stimulates the reproductive system, thereby increasing stamina. Reshapes the thighs and waist.

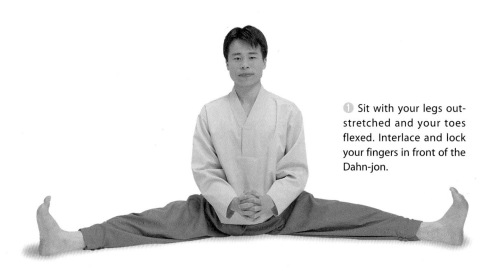

❶ Sit with your legs outstretched and your toes flexed. Interlace and lock your fingers in front of the Dahn-jon.

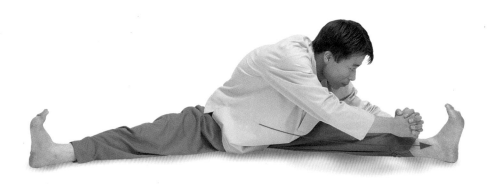

❷ Slowly move your body with a grinding motion towards the left toes and follow this movement with your eyes.

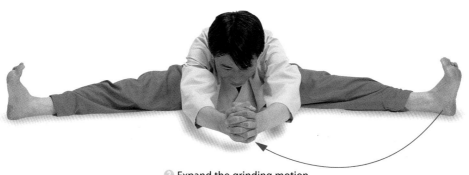

❸ Expand the grinding motion and slowly bring your body to the center, parallel to your Dahn-jon.

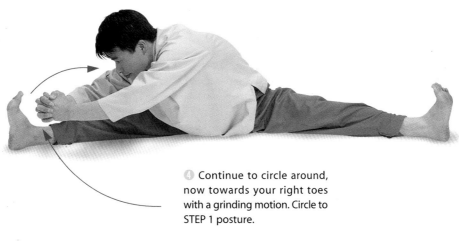

❹ Continue to circle around, now towards your right toes with a grinding motion. Circle to STEP 1 posture.

❺ Repeat three times. Continue to the opposite side.

4. SUPERMAN POSTURE VARIATION

Benefits This motion reshapes the back and waist. It is recommended to perform this exercise as soon as you awaken in the morning.

TIPS When you lift your arms and legs, proceed very slowly and with only few repetitions, not exceeding ten times in the beginning.

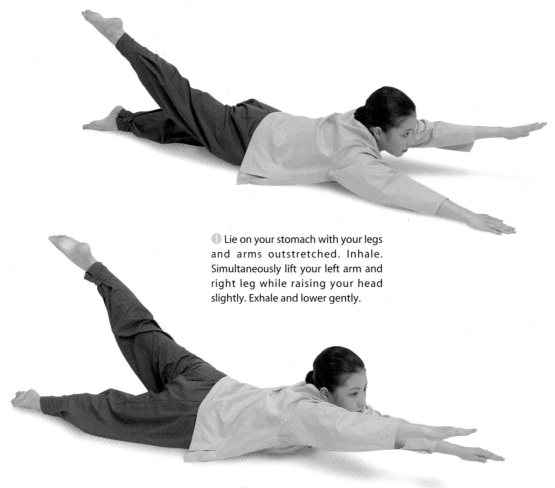

① Lie on your stomach with your legs and arms outstretched. Inhale. Simultaneously lift your left arm and right leg while raising your head slightly. Exhale and lower gently.

② Inhale and now raise your right arm and your left leg while raising your head slightly. Repeat five times.

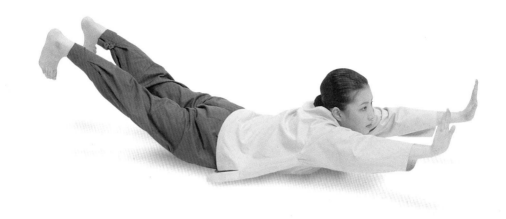

❸ Inhale. Simultaneously lift both arms and legs very gently with only your Dahn-jon touching the floor.

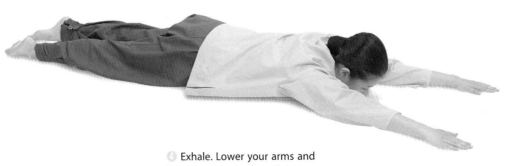

❹ Exhale. Lower your arms and legs gently to the floor. Relax.

5. HEAD ROTATION

Benefits Releases tension from the muscles in the neck. Reshapes the muscles in the neck. Enhances the quality of the voice.

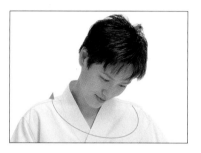

❶ Stand, or sit in a half-lotus postion. Begin very slowly to rotate your head with a circular motion in a 360-degree rotation. Then repeat to the other side.

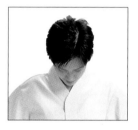 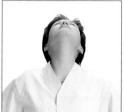 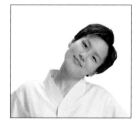 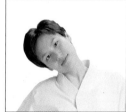

❷ Slowly move your head towards your chest and back and then towards the right shoulder and then to the left shoulder.

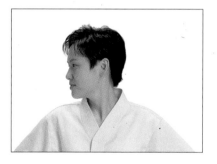 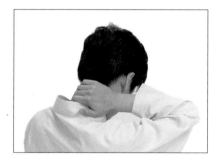

❸ Inhale. Sit still. Turn your head to the left very slowly. Hold it for a few seconds and then exhale to the center. Repeat to the right side. Repeat five times.

❹ Massage the back of your neck with your right hand and then alternate with your left hand.

6. LIFTING THE NECK WITH CLASPED HANDS

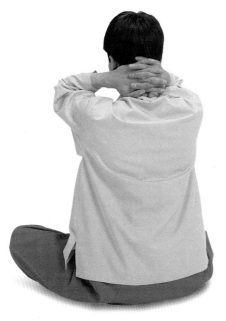

❶ Interlace and lock your fingers behind your neck.

❷ Gently tilt your head back while lifting your neck. Slowly release. Repeat four to five times.

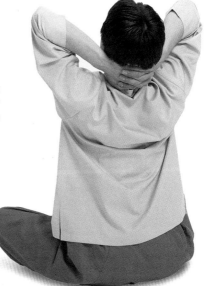

7. SIT-UP VARIATION

Benefits Reshapes abdominal muscles.

TIPS It is important to practice this exercise consistently to achieve maximum benefit. When you come to the lifting position, proceed cautiously using your entire upper body. Make certain that you do not bounce or exert undo effort with your shoulders. Maintain focus on your abdominal muscles to assist you while lifting. If the recommended thirty repetitions are too difficult, then begin with only a few repetitions and increase as you consistently practice.

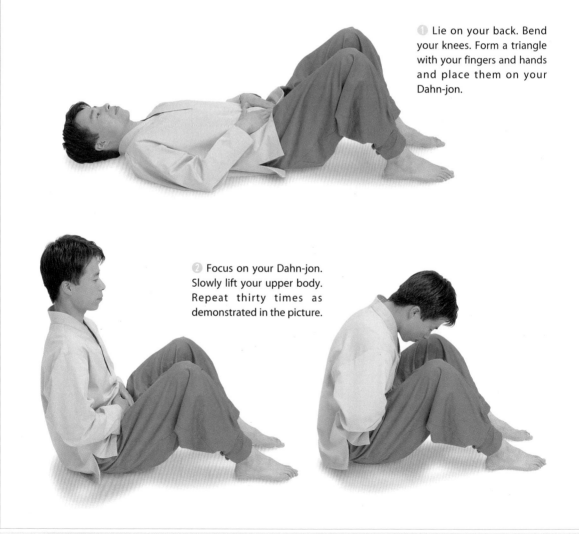

① Lie on your back. Bend your knees. Form a triangle with your fingers and hands and place them on your Dahn-jon.

② Focus on your Dahn-jon. Slowly lift your upper body. Repeat thirty times as demonstrated in the picture.

8. ANKLE JOINT EXERCISE

Benefits Effects shapely appearance of the ankles.

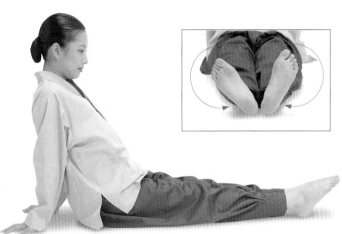

① Assume a sitting posture with your legs comfortably outstretched in front of you. Place your hands on the floor behind you with your fingers facing away. Slowly rotate your ankles 360-degrees alternating the direction of your movement.

② Extend one foot while simultaneously flexing the other foot, like a peddling motion. Change directions and continue with this movement.

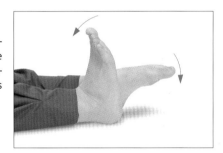

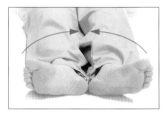

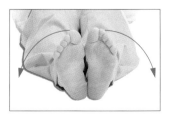

③ Keep your heels touching while you tap your toes together. Repeat one hundred times.

2) POOR EYESIGHT

As stress and tension increase through intensive and prolonged visual participation, the musculo-skeletal system associated with eye function becomes reactive causing such symptoms as headache, dizziness, gastrointestinal problems, blurry vision, redness in the eyes, pain in the eyeball, neck, shoulders, and back, and photosensitivity.

Adherents and practitioners of Eastern Medicine highlight the examination of the eyes routinely to signal the corresponding functioning of the major organs, particularly the liver and the kidneys. Surrounding the eye are nerves and meridian channels. To sustain the strength of the eyes, it is important to fortify the liver and kidneys and supply oxygen and Ki energy to the nerves that nourish the eyes.

The recommended Dahnhak Meridian exercises include techniques to stimulate the eyes, such as massage. It is extremely helpful to massage cervical vertebrae. This will relieve tension, fatigue and toxic stress from the system so as not to disturb the delicate balancing of the musculo-skeletal system and your vision. These exercises will also focus on building and sustaining Ki energy flow in the liver and kidneys to augment this process.

SENDING KI ENERGY TO EYES
(Book 2, p. 61)

Benefits Reduces redness in the eyes and helps to maintain visual acuity. Relieves fatigue from the eyes and helps them to look vibrant and healthy.

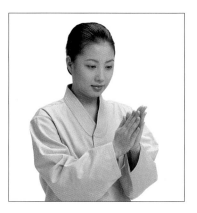

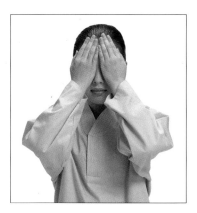

1. APPLYING PRESSURE AROUND EYES

TIPS   When people experience problems with their vision, it is important to see whether in fact these difficulties are related to a deficiency or imbalance of Ki energy in the liver, kidneys, and/or the heart. The Dahnhak Meridian exercises recommended in this section are particularly beneficial in balancing the Ki energy in these organs.

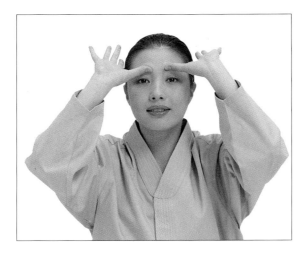

❶ With your thumbs or index fingers, gently press around the circumference of the eyes.

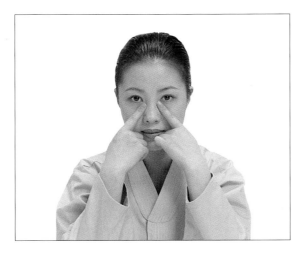

❷ With your index fingers, gently press the area under the eyes and around the bridge of the nose.

2. ROTATING EYEBALLS

Benefits Can help to improve vision.

METHOD Imagine looking straight ahead and viewing a triangle. Your eyeballs will gaze to look at each of the three points.

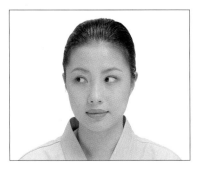 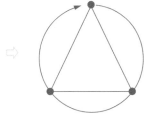

① Do not move your head while performing this exercise. Rotate only your eyes to follow the triangle. Rotate thirty-six times in one direction and then repeat thirty-six times in the other direction.

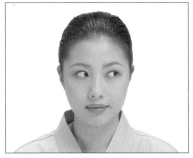 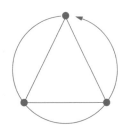

HELPFUL EXERCISES TO MAXIMIZE YOUR VISION

① On a sheet of paper, draw a bullet. Position yourself at a twenty inch distance. Maintain the gaze of your eyes on the bullet without blinking.

② After gazing for a while at the bullet, you will notice a white halo forming around the bullet. Keep focusing on the bullet while maintaining the distinct halo.

③ You may notice redness and teardrops from your eyes in the beginning of this exercise. Continue to keep your eyes open.

④ Now blink your eyes quickly thirty-six times. Then, close your eyes and relax. When you first perform this exercise, begin by gazing at the bullet for one minute. Then continue to progress to gazing at the bullet for up to five minutes.

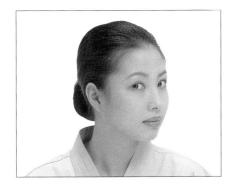 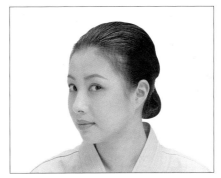

❷ Look at an imaginary bullet ahead of you. Now move your head to the right, while simultaneously maintaining your eyes straight ahead, gazing at the bullet. Hold for six seconds. Bring your head to the center for two seconds. Repeat to the other side.

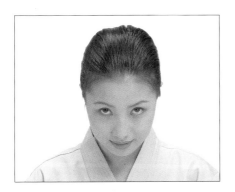 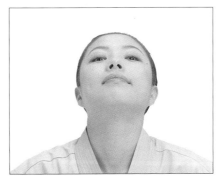

❸ Look at an imaginary bullet ahead of you. Move your head down towards your chest while maintaining the gaze of your eyes on the bullet straight ahead of you. While still gazing at the bullet straight ahead, now move your head backward towards your neck. Keep your eyes open throughout this exercise.

3) IMPAIRED HEARING

✿

Our ears, as opposed to other sense organs, move the least when we exercise. At about age twenty, ear problems can begin to occur and hearing can progressively become impaired. Later on, tinnitus, or the sensation of ringing in the ears, can occur. This condition can be extremely irritating. There can be a variety of causes, including cardio-vascular problems, earwax, endocronological problems, or exposure to high pitched sounds over a period of time.

The ear has about two-hundred acupressure points correlated with our body functioning. When you experience problems with your ears, it is important to strengthen the Ki energy in the kidneys. The recommended Dahnhak Meridian exercises in this section highlight exercises that are beneficial to maximizing Ki energy flow in the kidneys to augment proper functioning of the ears.

1. STIMULATING THE CHUN-GO ACUPRESSURE POINTS

Benefits By stimulating the Chun-go acupressure points located behind the ear, the stagnant energy around the ears dissipates, thereby strengthening the nerves around the ears. It can help to improve hearing and help reduce ringing in the ears.

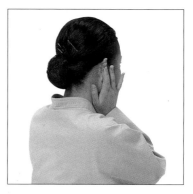

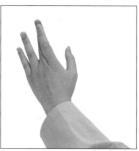

Place your index finger on the top of your middle finger. Use the middle finger, with the index finger still on top of the middle finger to close the flap of your ear, and cover the opening of the ear. With a snapping motion, move the index finger off the middle finger and tap your bone behind your ear with the index finger. Repeat this swift motion to match the number of your age. When you perform this motion swiftly, you will hear the sound of a drum.

2. EAR PRESSING AND RELEASING WITH PALMS

① Cover your ears with your palms. Relax your mouth and keep it slightly ajar. Apply gentle pressure. Slowly count to three and release quickly.

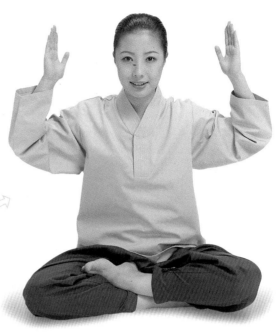

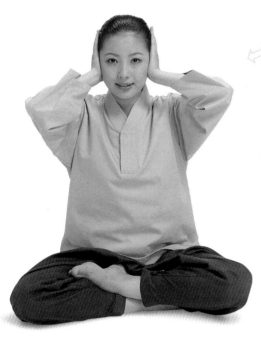

② Repeat five times. Massage your ears. Then, with your thumbs and index fingers, gently pull on your ears in all directions to stimulate the acupressure points.

PRESSING THE CHUN-JU ACUPRESSURE POINTS (Book 1, p. 34)

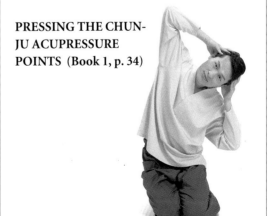

4) INSOMNIA

Insomnia arises from an imbalance of Ki and blood circulation throughout the body, whereby it becomes blocked in the head and presses on the brain. Vulnerability to insomnia can come about when there is continual stress, excessive thinking about worrisome issues, trauma, or shock, thereby compromising the body's immune system. According to adherents of Eastern Medicine, the principle of Su-Seung-Hwa-Gang (water energy up and fire energy down, see page 32, book 1) is the requisite condition for a healthy body, mind, and spirit. When the body is not adequately rested, and/or is undergoing intense stress, Su-Seung-Hwa-Gang is thwarted and the reverse occurs; that is fire energy now goes up towards the head, and water energy travels down towards the lower abdomen. Some of the symptoms that may occur are redness in the face, shoulder pain, and pain in the middle of the chest along the Im-maek, signaling blockage in this area.

The recommended Dahnhak Meridian exercises in this section emphasize relaxation and optimize the Su-Seung-Hwa-Gang flow, which is crucial in alleviating Insomnia.

BODY TAPPING (Book 1, p. 22)

Benefits Enhances blood and Ki energy circulation throughout the body and releases stagnant energy. Strengthens and activates the cells and nervous system as it helps to alleviate the problem of insomnia.

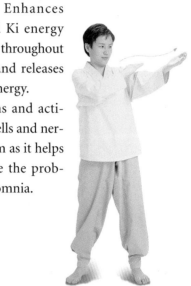

SOLE CLAPPING (Book 2, p. 21)

Benefits Stimulates the feet and legs and helps to augment the flow of fire energy down to the lower abdomen.

TIPS When you perform this exercise, relax your knee joints as you clap your feet.

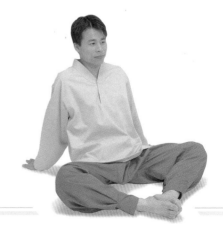

1. QUIETING THE MIND THROUGH FOCUSING ON YOUR INNER SELF

Benefits Helps to bring fire energy towards the lower abdomen for further relaxation of the body and mind.

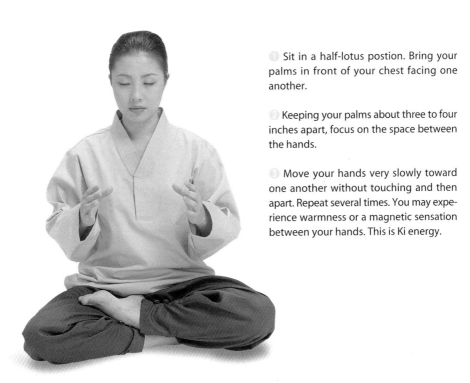

① Sit in a half-lotus postion. Bring your palms in front of your chest facing one another.

② Keeping your palms about three to four inches apart, focus on the space between the hands.

③ Move your hands very slowly toward one another without touching and then apart. Repeat several times. You may experience warmness or a magnetic sensation between your hands. This is Ki energy.

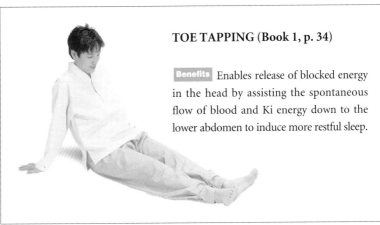

TOE TAPPING (Book 1, p. 34)

Benefits Enables release of blocked energy in the head by assisting the spontaneous flow of blood and Ki energy down to the lower abdomen to induce more restful sleep.

2. WHOLE BODY RELAXATION

Benefits This exercise is especially helpful for the conditions of heart disease, hypertension, insomnia, and headaches.

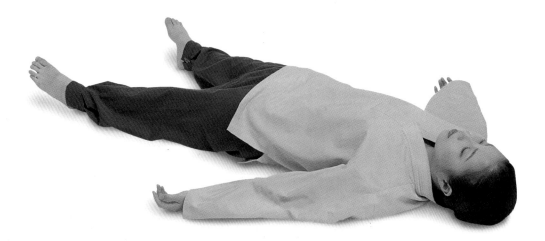

① Lie comfortably on your back, with feet shoulder width apart and arms at about forty-five degrees from the body. Close your eyes.

② Inhale slowly, deeply and comfortably. Exhale slowly and release tension from the body. Repeat three times.

③ As your eyes remain closed, begin to imagine in your mind's eye that you are observing yourself with clear focus. You see all the parts of your body from the top of your head down to the tips of your toes.

④ Continue to imagine that your head is becoming more and more clear and cool.

⑤ Relax your facial muscles. Begin to form a gentle smile. With your mind's eye, observe your smiling face.

⑥ Relax your neck and shoulders. Imagine that stagnant energy is moving from your neck and shoulders out through your fingertips.

⑦ Focus on your chest. Feel your chest begin to expand along with your breathing. Imagine your chest feeling cool and comfortable.

⑧ With your mind's eye, observe your waist and abdominal area, your thighs, knees, legs, ankles, and toes. As you continue to focus on your breathing and release tension, feel the comfort and quiet around these areas.

⑨ As you become more and more relaxed, imagine your body feeling heavier and heavier.

⑩ Continue to breathe normally. Now, as you exhale, feel your body begin to sink deeper and deeper into the earth as you become more and more relaxed.

⑪ Imagine a very special place of peace, tranquility, and comfort just for you, provided by the whole universe.

3. STANDING THIGH STRETCH AND BALANCING

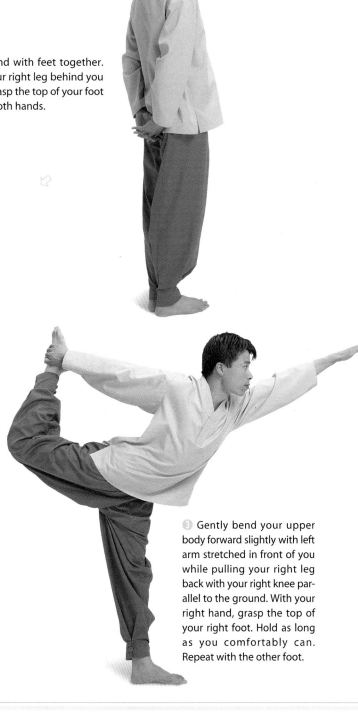

❶ Stand with feet together. Lift your right leg behind you and grasp the top of your foot with both hands.

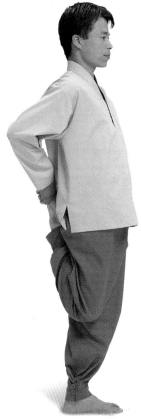

❷ Gently, pull the top of the foot towards your hip. Repeat ten times.

❸ Gently bend your upper body forward slightly with left arm stretched in front of you while pulling your right leg back with your right knee parallel to the ground. With your right hand, grasp the top of your right foot. Hold as long as you comfortably can. Repeat with the other foot.

4. OPENING THE IM-MAEK

Benefits This exercise will help to release stagnant fire energy from the chest that has become blocked. It is beneficial for insomnia and headaches.

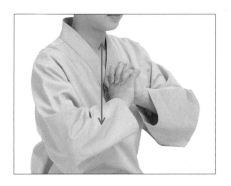

① Sit in a half-lotus postion or stand. Interlace your fingers and begin to gently tap up and down from the throat area to the chest.

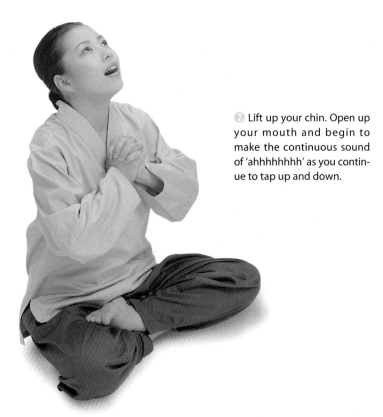

② Lift up your chin. Open up your mouth and begin to make the continuous sound of 'ahhhhhhhh' as you continue to tap up and down.

5. BRIDGE POSTURE VARIATION

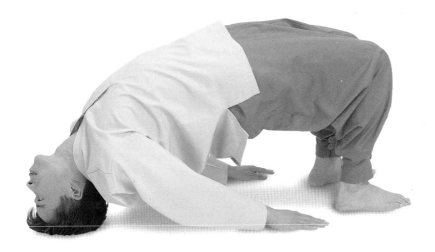

① Lie on your back. Bend your knees. Inhale. Lift your hips and raise your chin up. Place your body weight on the top of your head. Hold for as long as you comfortably can.

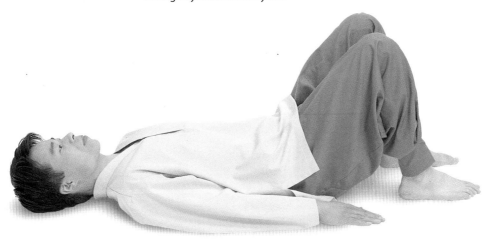

② Continue to hold this posture until you begin to feel your face flush. Quickly drop your hips and waist down to the floor, while at the same time making the sound 'hoht.' Repeat three times.

6. BUTTOCK TAPPING WITH HEELS

Benefits Assists in circulating blood from the lower extremities to the head. Will cool the head and calm the mind.

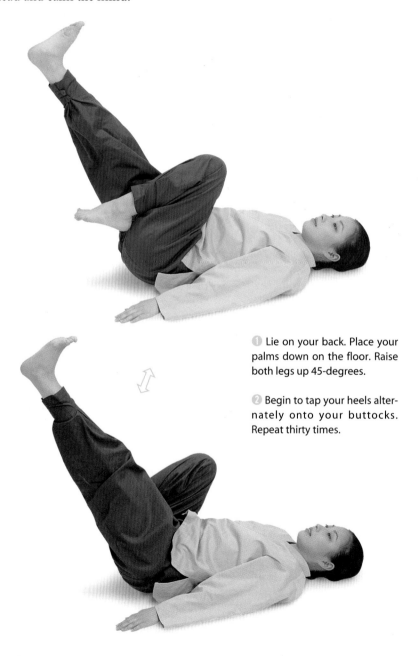

① Lie on your back. Place your palms down on the floor. Raise both legs up 45-degrees.

② Begin to tap your heels alternately onto your buttocks. Repeat thirty times.

7. ROTATING ANKLES WITH HANDS

Benefits Relaxes waist and legs. Enables blood and Ki energy to circulate throughout the body.

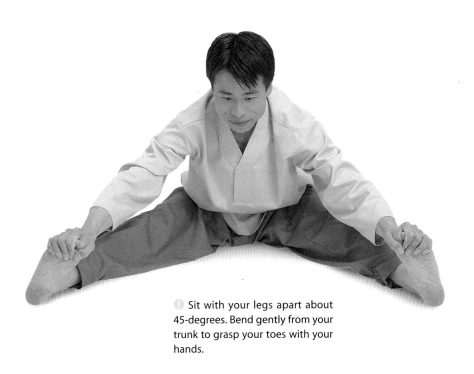

① Sit with your legs apart about 45-degrees. Bend gently from your trunk to grasp your toes with your hands.

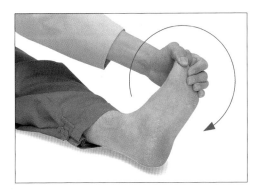

② Rotate in a circular manner, first inward and then outward.

5) HANGOVERS

When people consume alcohol, there is a noticeable smell emanating from their breath. Oftentimes, there is an accompanying headache. Eventually the alcohol evaporates and the smell dissipates. It is important to release the toxins from the body caused by the alcohol as quickly as possible.

Dahn-jon breathing is not advised after generous consumption of alcohol. In its effort to filter the toxins from the body, the liver, already weakened by stress and fatigue, is further taxed as it attempts to detoxify the effects of the alcohol. Dahn-jon breathing causes an increase in the circulation of the alcohol throughout the body, causing more effort for the liver to detoxify the body. Instead, it is recommended to perform deep breathing, accompanied by Meridian exercises in this section. This will open the liver meridian channels to enhance blood circulation and the metabolic system, thus assisting in the detoxification from the effects of the alcohol.

BODY TAPPING
(Book 1, p. 22)

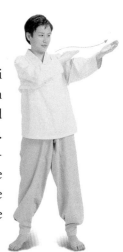

Benefits Enhances Ki and blood circulation throughout the body and releases stagnant toxins. Helps eliminate insomnia and strengthens the nervous system and the cells throughout the body.

SOLE CLAPPING
(Book 2, p. 21)

Benefits Stimulates the feet and legs as it brings fire energy towards the lower abdomen.

TIPS Relax your knees and keep them soft to avoid compression around the knee joints.

SIDE BEND WITH LOCKED FINGERS
(Book 2, p. 57)

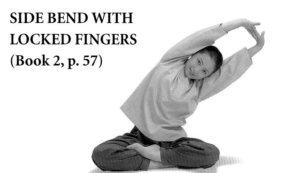

1. DEEP BREATHING

Benefits Enables quick alcohol evaporation from the blood stream.

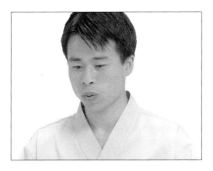

Inhale slowly and deeply through your nose to the lower abdomen. Exhale slowly and completely through your mouth. Repeat this ten times.

2. OPENING MERIDIANS IN THE LEGS

Benefits This motion will open the Liver and Gall Bladder Meridians and enhance liver and gall bladder functioning. This will help to quickly detoxify the alcohol from the body.

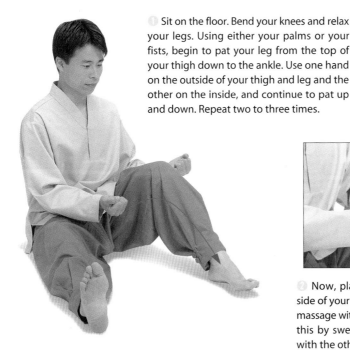

① Sit on the floor. Bend your knees and relax your legs. Using either your palms or your fists, begin to pat your leg from the top of your thigh down to the ankle. Use one hand on the outside of your thigh and leg and the other on the inside, and continue to pat up and down. Repeat two to three times.

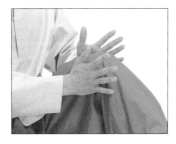

② Now, place your palms on either side of your knees and begin to gently massage with a circular motion. Follow this by sweeping downward. Repeat with the other leg.

3. CHEST OPENING

TIPS Keep your elbows at a 90-degree angle when performing this exercise.

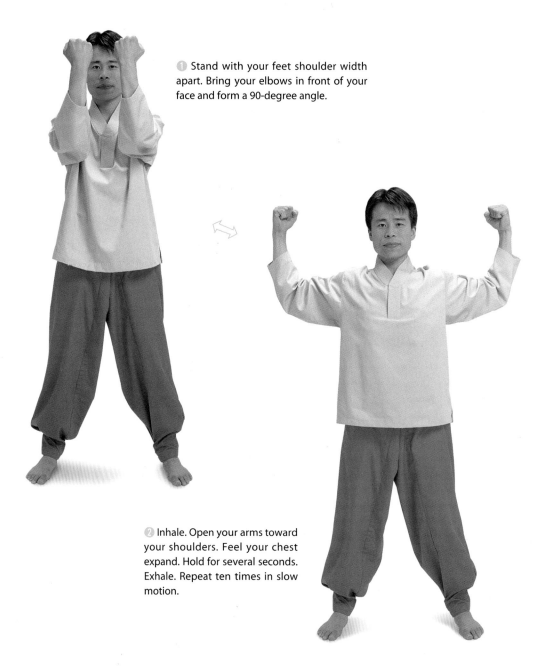

① Stand with your feet shoulder width apart. Bring your elbows in front of your face and form a 90-degree angle.

② Inhale. Open your arms toward your shoulders. Feel your chest expand. Hold for several seconds. Exhale. Repeat ten times in slow motion.

4. SIDE LEG LIFT FOR LIVER

Benefits Enhances the Liver and Gall Bladder Meridian functioning to enable rapid evaporation of alcohol toxins from the body. Helps lessen fatigue.

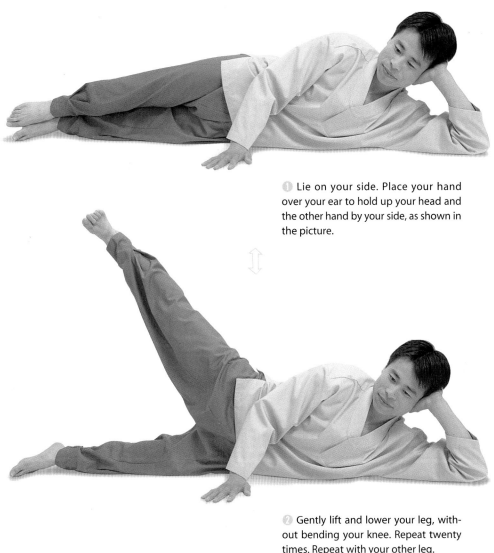

❶ Lie on your side. Place your hand over your ear to hold up your head and the other hand by your side, as shown in the picture.

❷ Gently lift and lower your leg, without bending your knee. Repeat twenty times. Repeat with your other leg.

5. PRESSING THE SPACE BETWEEN THE RIBS

Benefits Open the chest, relieving fatigue in the liver and tightness in the chest.

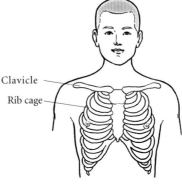

Clavicle

Rib cage

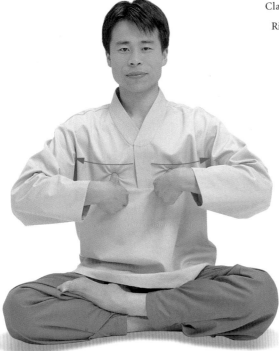

❶ Beginning with the space between the clavicle and the top of the rib, press with your thumbs beginning with the center and then continue outward to the sides. Press again with your thumbs from the center in the space between the bones of the ribs, proceeding downward towards the bottom of the rib cage.

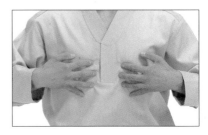

❷ Place all your fingers between the bones of the ribs. Exhale, and simultaneously press in the spaces between your ribs. Continue this motion, making certain to cover the spaces between your entire rib cage.

6. SPINE TWISTING

Benefits This posture will stimulate the Tenth Thoracic Vertebrae to enhance liver and kidney function. Detoxifies, as it enables more rapid excretion of water from the body.

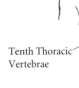

Tenth Thoracic
Vertebrae

Sit on the floor. Allow your left knee to stand on the floor, while bending your right knee on the floor under your left knee, as shown in the picture.

Grasp the outside of your left ankle by placing your right arm over the left knee.

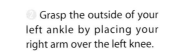

Inhale while maintaining a straight, but not rigid spine. Turn your upper body to the left and follow with the gaze of your eyes. Focus on your spine. Exhale and gently turn again towards center.

Repeat on the other side. Repeat this exercise three times.

5. OTHER CONDITIONS

6) LETHARGY/FATIGUE

Chronic fatigue can result from lack of sleep, overwork, malnutrition, excessive stress, liver disease, or fatty deposits in the liver, impeding proper Ki circulation, which is vital for the health of the person. People will oftentimes find that even if they rest, they will still feel fatigue. Symptoms such as pain and stiffness, particularly in the neck, shoulders, and lower back, and a general heaviness in the body signal to adherents of Eastern Medicine that blockages in the acupressure points and meridians are causing these symptoms.

The recommended Dahnhak Meridian exercises in this section will help to release the stagnant Ki energy that has become blocked, revitalizing energy, and reducing fatigue.

SWEEPING DOWN THE BLADDER MERIDIAN (Book 1, p. 99)

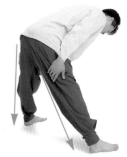

Benefits Stimulates the Bladder Meridian as it quickly relieves fatigue from waist and legs.

THIGH STRETCH (Book 1, p. 129)

Benefits Enables fire energy to come down to the lower abdomen to enable more peaceful and restful sleep.

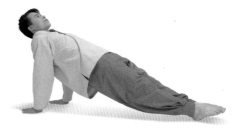

BICYCLE EXERCISE (Book 1, p. 142)

Benefits Strengthens lower extremities and stimulates the muscles and nerves around the perineal and reproductive glands. Enhances stamina; enables more effective blood and Ki energy circulation in the head. Relieves fatigue from the lower extremities.

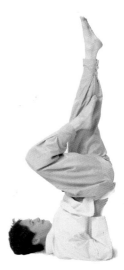

BOW POSTURE (Book 2, p. 74)

Benefits Stimulates the spine and the central nervous system, realigns the spine, and enhances the function of the endocrine glands. Speeds recovery from chronic general fatigue. Beneficial for those spending prolonged hours sitting or in other sedentary positions.

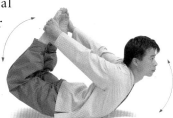

OPENING MERIDIAN CHANNELS IN THE LEGS (Book 2, p. 165)

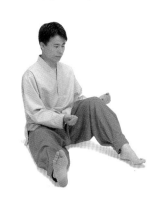

1. STRETCHING ARMS TO THE SKY

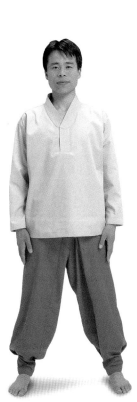

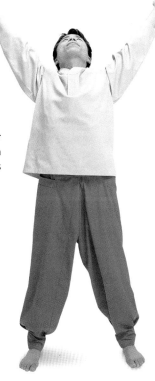

① Stand with your legs shoulder width apart with your arms down at your sides.

② Inhale. Keeping fingers together, expand your chest as you stretch your arms above your head, towards the sky. Keep your elbows soft, but not bent. Your weight should be felt on your toes.

③ Exhale to STEP 1, and repeat once more.

2. PUSHING ENERGY WITH THE HANDS TOWARDS THE SKY AND THE EARTH

Benefits Helps recover from fatigue as the strong energy from heaven and earth is received in the body.

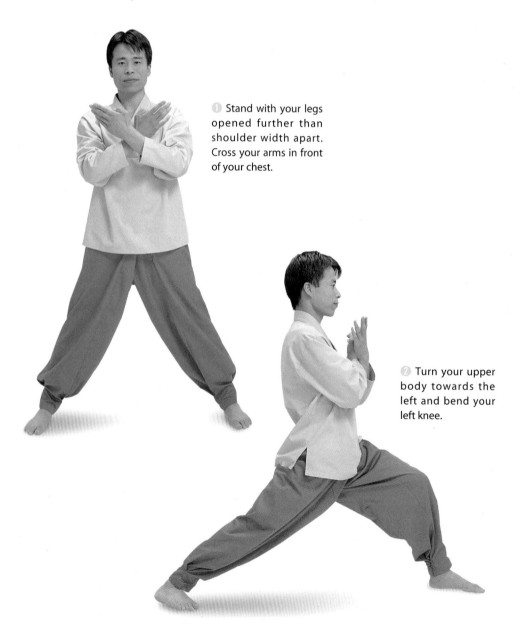

① Stand with your legs opened further than shoulder width apart. Cross your arms in front of your chest.

② Turn your upper body towards the left and bend your left knee.

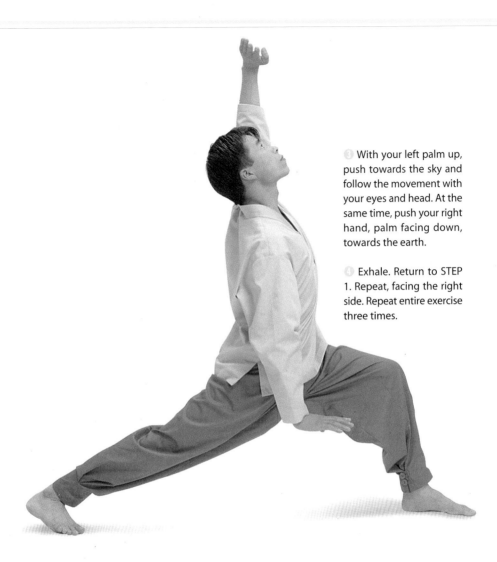

③ With your left palm up, push towards the sky and follow the movement with your eyes and head. At the same time, push your right hand, palm facing down, towards the earth.

④ Exhale. Return to STEP 1. Repeat, facing the right side. Repeat entire exercise three times.

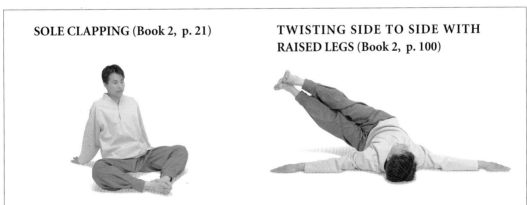

SOLE CLAPPING (Book 2, p. 21)

TWISTING SIDE TO SIDE WITH RAISED LEGS (Book 2, p. 100)

7) SPRING FATIGUE

People will often notice that as the spring season approaches, they are very fatigued and not as energetic as they would like to be. Adherents of Eastern Medicine believe this is due to the fluctuation in the bio-rhythms of the body. As the body temperatures rise in spring time in response to the changes in atmospheric temperature, muscles begin to relax, and the meridians open with more ease to the entire peripheral area. This allows more vital Ki energy and blood circulation flow. In the winter time, however, muscles are more contracted. Ki energy and blood circulation flow are more constricted. In the change from winter to spring, the organs need more energy, as they increase their functioning capacity with the change of season. People who are sedentary and do not participate in appropriate exercise for the body have less Ki energy accumulated during the winter season. They will find it even more arduous to adjust to the change of season, and can experience significant spring fatigue.

The most significant symptoms signaling spring fatigue are: lethargy, decrease in appetite, digestive problems, and dizziness. The Dahnhak Meridian exercises recommended in this section are designed to enable increased vitality and augment the shift to the spring season.

TIP-TOE STRETCHING
(Book 2, p. 97)

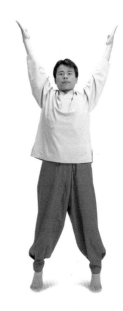

PUSHING ENERGY WITH HANDS TOWARDS THE SKY AND THE EARTH (Book 2, p. 172)

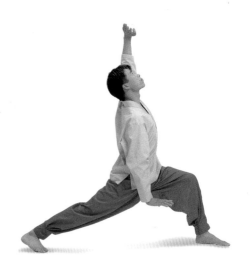

1. PUSHING KI ENERGY

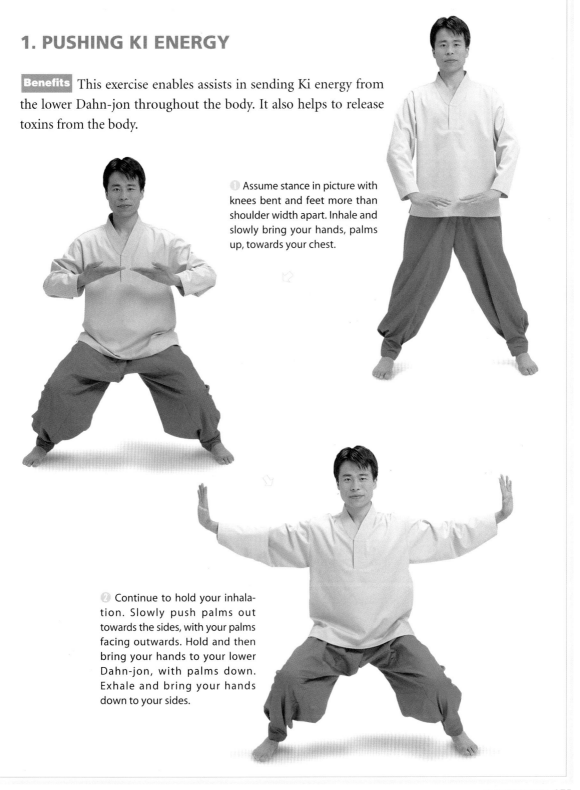

Benefits This exercise enables assists in sending Ki energy from the lower Dahn-jon throughout the body. It also helps to release toxins from the body.

① Assume stance in picture with knees bent and feet more than shoulder width apart. Inhale and slowly bring your hands, palms up, towards your chest.

② Continue to hold your inhalation. Slowly push palms out towards the sides, with your palms facing outwards. Hold and then bring your hands to your lower Dahn-jon, with palms down. Exhale and bring your hands down to your sides.

2. STRETCHING WHILE FORMING CIRCLES

Benefits Enhances functioning of the organs. Helps release stagnant blood from the abdomen and facilitate Ki energy flow.

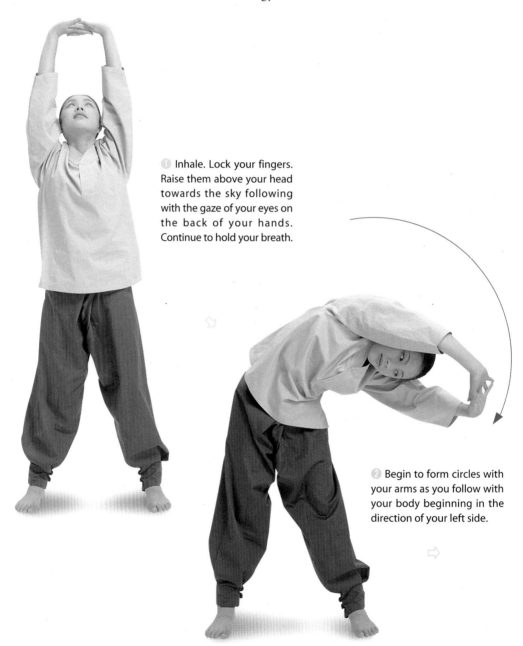

① Inhale. Lock your fingers. Raise them above your head towards the sky following with the gaze of your eyes on the back of your hands. Continue to hold your breath.

② Begin to form circles with your arms as you follow with your body beginning in the direction of your left side.

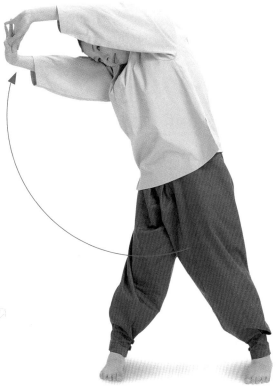

④ Complete the circle while bringing arms towards the right side.

⑤ Exhale. Unlock your fingers. Repeat the motion of forming circles beginning on your right side. Repeat twice to the right and left sides.

③ Continue to form circles touching the floor with your palms as you reach the center of the circle.

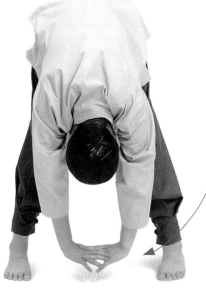

3. SITTING HAM-STRING STRETCH

TIPS This exercise will achieve its benefits if you remember to keep your knee straight but soft during the stretch and bend your head back as in the picture on the bottom of the page for STEPs 3 and 4.

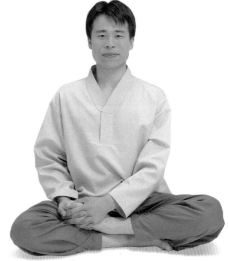

① Sit on the floor or on a chair. With your left hand, grasp the bottom of your left foot.

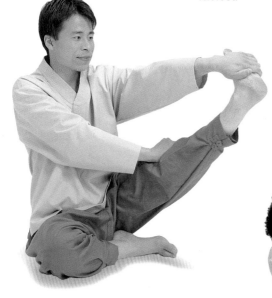

② Place your right hand on your left knee with slight pressure as you gently begin to stretch your left leg with foot flexed as shown in the center picture.

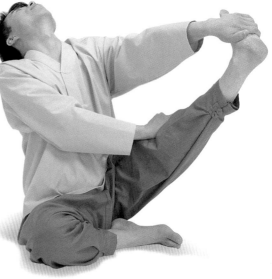

③ With your left leg straight but soft, gently tilt your head backwards following with the gaze of your eyes.

④ Repeat this exercise with your right leg. Perform this stretch two more times with each leg.

4. FORWARD BEND WITH CLASPED HANDS

TIPS   Keep your knees straight but soft. When you bend your upper body, straighten your arms without locking them as you bring them forward.

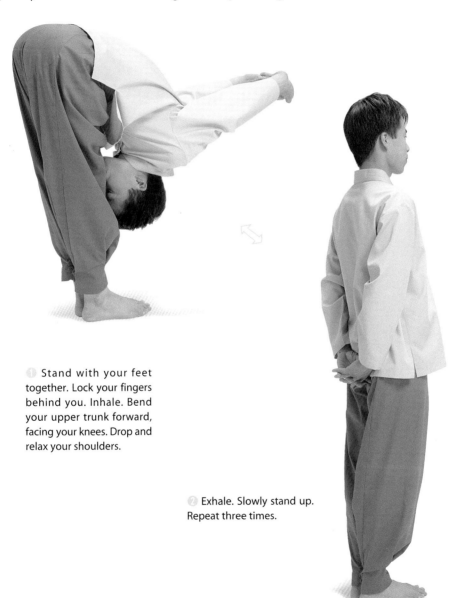

① Stand with your feet together. Lock your fingers behind you. Inhale. Bend your upper trunk forward, facing your knees. Drop and relax your shoulders.

② Exhale. Slowly stand up. Repeat three times.

KI ENERGY BRINGS
HEALTH TO THE BODY
AND PEACE TO THE MIND

APPENDIX

1. THE SPINE, MAIN PILLAR OF OUR BODY

The spinal column, pillar of the human body, consists of seven cervical vertebrae, twelve thoracic vertebrae, five lumbar vertebrae, the sacrum (five fused vertebrae) and the coccyx (four fused vertebrae) in descending order. The entire spinal column, which consists of thirty-three vertebrae, is S-shaped. Since autonomic nerves corresponding to each organ travel throughout the spinal column, problems in the spine have an impact on the related organs.

There are disks between cervical vertebrae, through which nerves travel. When problems arise in the cervical vertebrae, they in turn put pressure on the nerves, which can cause pain anywhere in the body. Nerves that branch out of the thoracic vertebrae connect to the five viscera (solid organs) and six entrails (hollow organs) and regulate functions of the internal organs. Therefore, problems in the thoracic vertebrae affect the internal organs.

If the crossbeam that supports the center of a house were to collapse, the house itself would collapse. Likewise, if the spine, the pillar of the

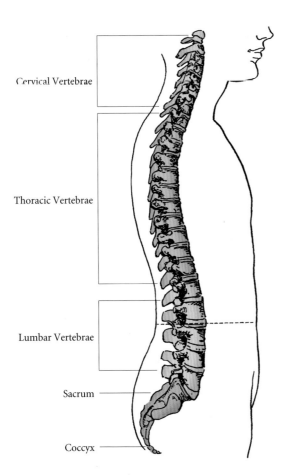

Cervical Vertebrae

Thoracic Vertebrae

Lumbar Vertebrae

Sacrum

Coccyx

human body, is injured, this compromises the entire body. The spine aligns the body and is the foundation of all our strength.

Poor posture and bad habits threaten health of the lower back and spine. For example, sitting with the hip pulled forward, sitting cross-legged, and talking on the phone with your head bent to one side, are all detrimental to your spine. It is important to form habits such as sitting with the spine straight, and making sure that your bend your knees when you lift a heavy item. When you do Dahnhak Meridian exercises regularly, it is possible to correct a misaligned spinal column with pulling and stretching movements.

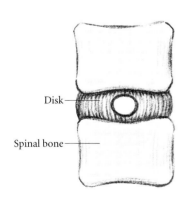

Disk

Spinal bone

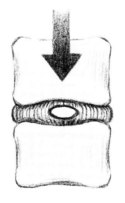

Violent movement, sudden shock, or poor posture can damage the disks in the spinal column. When this occurs, the damaged disk may exert pressure on the nerves, causing pain and inhibiting movement of the spine itself.

Normal disk   **Disk deformed by pressure**

2. POSITION OF ORGANS AND THE SKELETON

Can you accurately point to where the stomach is located in body? Is the liver located on the right, or the left side? Understanding the body's structure and functions, including position of the organs and skeleton is helpful when doing Dahnhak Meridian exercises.

When you send energy to a specific organ or a problem area, the more accurately you can imagine the position or the shape of the organ, the greater the effect will be. When you execute Meridian exercises, you should wholeheartedly appreciate and be thankful for these hard-working organs.

The liver is the chemical factory of our body, the stomach is a factory where food is broken down and processed and the heart is a pump that circulates blood throughout the whole body. When you do Meridian exercises, you should wholeheartedly thank and cherish these hard-working organs.

Bones support the body and protect the internal organs. The skull protects the brain and the ribs encircle the heart and lungs. Bone marrow generates red blood cells that deliver oxygen and nutrients to the body and white blood cells to destroy harmful bacteria. When your body moves, you should focus on each movement. Begin observing your body and later you will observe your mind. In other words, we can reach the mind through the body. The body is a mirror of the mind and the dwelling place of ther soul.

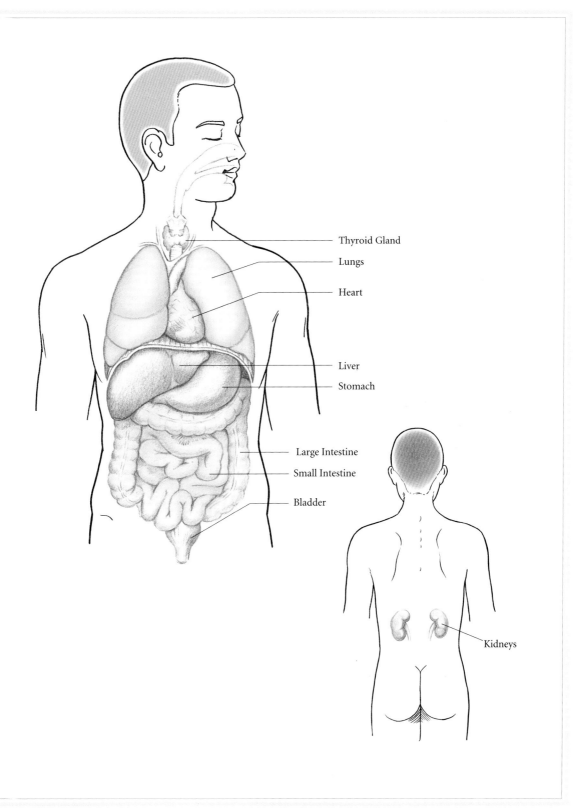

Thyroid Gland

Lungs

Heart

Liver

Stomach

Large Intestine

Small Intestine

Bladder

Kidneys

3. MERIDIANS, RIVERS OF KI ENERGY

Meridians and acupressure points are an invisible network of life. Meridians or channels are the pathways through which Ki energy travels through the body. There are 365 primary acupressure points and 12 primary meridians in the human body. Acupressure points are like train stations where Ki energy collects, and meridians are the tracks connecting these points. The 12 primary meridians or channels are Lung, Large intestine, Stomach, Spleen, Heart, Small Intestine, Urinary Bladder, Kidney, Pericardium, Triple Burner, Gall Bladder, and Liver. They travel bilaterally in the right and left sides of the body.

Disease is created because the flow of Ki energy that travels through meridians and acupressure points is blocked somewhere. It is similar to a traffic jam when roads are inoperative. The acupressure points and the meridians are intergral parts of the entire body. Even the sole of the foot is connected to every organ of the body.

As few as nine, to more than sixty acupressure points are distributed along a single meridian, but you don't have to memorize all of them. Understanding the general flow of a meridian is a great help to your practice. For example, when you have problems in the liver, simply tapping, massaging, applying pressure, or stroking along the liver meridian will be highly effective. If you practice long enough, you will sense electricity or a sense of pressure along the meridians, therefore without memorizing the positions of all of the acupressure points, you know where they are.

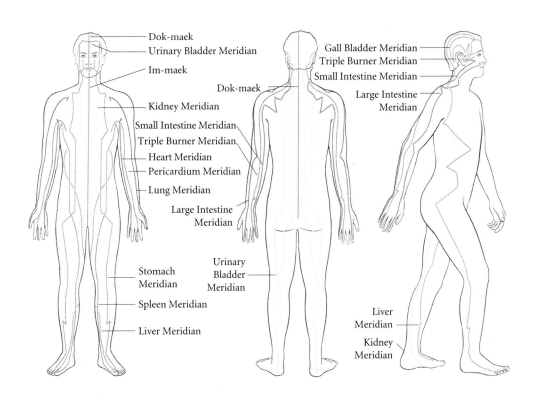

Dok-maek
Urinary Bladder Meridian
Im-maek
Kidney Meridian
Small Intestine Meridian
Triple Burner Meridian
Heart Meridian
Pericardium Meridian
Lung Meridian
Large Intestine Meridian
Stomach Meridian
Spleen Meridian
Liver Meridian

Dok-maek
Urinary Bladder Meridian

Gall Bladder Meridian
Triple Burner Meridian
Small Intestine Meridian
Large Intestine Meridian

Liver Meridian
Kidney Meridian

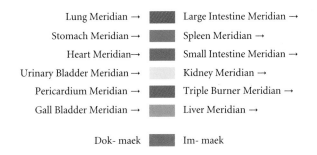

Lung Meridian →   Large Intestine Meridian →
Stomach Meridian →   Spleen Meridian →
Heart Meridian→   Small Intestine Meridian →
Urinary Bladder Meridian →   Kidney Meridian →
Pericardium Meridian →   Triple Burner Meridian →
Gall Bladder Meridian →   Liver Meridian →

Dok- maek   Im- maek

1) For difficulty breathing, asthma, and tightness in the chest

Lung Meridian

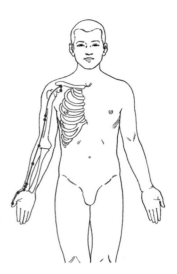

When the lungs, which assimilate air and distribute oxygen to the five viscera weaken, the flow of the Lung Meridian is easily blocked. When there are problems in the Lung Meridian, the function of all respiratory organs(nose, throat, lungs and bronchi) will be impaired as well. You may experience a hot face, dry mouth, stifling feeling in the chest, aching arms and legs, and sweaty palms. As the function of the lungs deteriorates, you may appear listless, and your skin may be dull. Under these conditions, applying pressure to the acupressure points along the Lung Meridian will facilitate the flow of energy and revitalize the organs.

2) When the white of the eye turns yellowish and the throat hurts

Large Intestine Meridian

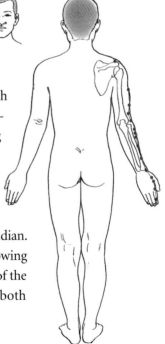

With toothache, stuffy nose, nosebleed, sore throat, or if the whites of the eyes turn yellowish, there may be a problem with the Large Intestine Meridian. You may have pain along the shoulders and arms, especially to the index fingers. In this case, pressing on the Chun-chu acupressure points, located on both sides of the navel, and the Dae-jang-yu acupressure points, behind the upper part of the pelvis, will be very sensitive. This signals dysfunction in the Large Intestine Meridian. In this case, give a finger pressure treatment along the flow of the Large Intestine Meridian. With your index finger pointed upward, stimulate to the wrist following the line of the index finger. Then follow up to the depressed point of the shoulders and lightly stimulate an area next to the airway on both sides.

3) For sores around the mouth, tension in the jaws, headache in the area of the eyes and sinuses or for pain in the abdominal region or the lateral aspect of the lower limbs

Stomach Meridian

Problems in the Stomach Meridian result in headache with severe pain, particularly in the forehead, around the eyes, and in the back of the head. Other symptoms include stuffy nose and occasional nosebleeds. There may also be sores around the mouth, sore throat, stomach cramps, and heavy and achy feeling in the legs from the thigh to the knee. Complexion and skin tone may become lusterless and dull. Lips may be dry, and articulation may be poor. In this case, the Jok-sam-ni tapping or toe tapping is beneficial. Also, relax and lightly tap along the Stomach Meridian from the side of the head, front of the ear, and the cheek in a straight line.

4) For nausea and frequent belching

Spleen Meridian

The spleen is mainly responsible for digestion. When the spleen functions harmoniously, digestion is good and there is abundant Ki energy and blood in the body. However, when the spleen is out of balance, you may experience a lack of Ki energy or insufficient blood in some or all parts of your body. You may have poor digestion that will lead to stomachache, diarrhea, and loss of appetite.

When the spleen is lethargic, your tongue may stiffen and you may feel pain and heaviness above the stomach. You may also feel nauseated and burp often. You may experience indigestion, frequent constipation, cold legs, and stiffness in the knees. Women may experience abnormal periods, occasional irregular uterine bleeding and insomnia. For these symptoms, it is beneficial to stimulate the Yong-chun acupressure points daily, and press the Spleen Meridian inside of the foot and the leg with your thumb.

5) For pain when pressing below the solar plexus, above the chest or upper part of the arm

Heart Meridian

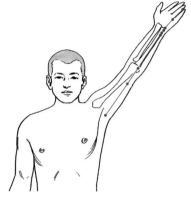

The Heart Meridian governs functioning of the heart and regulates brain function. Bloodshot eyes, a dry throat and insomnia are indications of problems with the heart. It may be painful under the solar plexus and there may be acute pain in the arms and little fingers. Those who have problems in the Heart Meridian usually have a flushed face. They generally have strong pulsation in the side of the head, the neck, wrists, top of the foot and the stomach. They may find it difficult to control their emotions and get easily fatigued. Under these condition, if you press below the solar plexus and inside of the shoulder blades, you will feel pain and may find swelling or lumps on palpation. For these symptoms, tap the depression between the breasts with your fingertips or fist and tap the Heart Mcridian, from the armpit, down the arm to to the little finger.

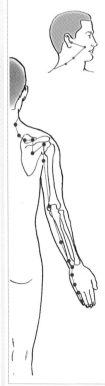

6) If the whites of the eye turns yellowish, hearing becomes dull, or with urinary difficulties

Small Intestine Meridian

The Small Intestine Meridian regulates functioning of the small intestine which is in charge of the absorption of nutrients. The small intestine acts as a filter between pure and stale energy, receiving food from the stomach and absorbing energy from the food following the digestive processes. During this process, pure energy transfers to the spleen and stale energy to the large intestine. Some fluids with stale energy go directly to the kidneys and bladder.

When you have problems with the small intestine, the whites of the eye become yellow and hearing becomes less acute. The cheeks may swell and the throat may be sore. The head can feel heavy and the arms ache or feel chilled. For these symptoms, apply finger pressure, with the top of the hands upward, on the area corresponding to the Small Intestine Meridian between the wrist and the root of the little finger, and on up the back of the arm.

7) The secret of youth is in the Urinary Bladder Meridian

Urinary Bladder Meridian

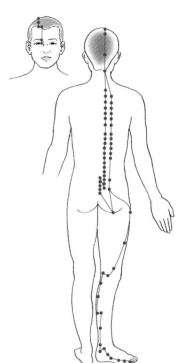

Problems with the Urinary Bladder Meridian include pain and tension in the occipital and neck area, fever and chills, nasal congestion, eye disease, low back pain, cramps in the backs of the legs and urinary difficulties. This meridian also affects reproductive functioning. Acupressure points along the sides of the spine are extremely important body reflex points that quickly signal problems arising in the internal organs. For menopausal symptoms or problems in the reproductive organs, regulate the Urinary Bladder Meridian. Stretch the legs forward and alternately shake each leg in a flop, or bend your upper body forward to activate the Urinary Bladder Meridian.

8) When the Kidney Meridian weakens, so does the lower back and knees.

Kidney Meridian

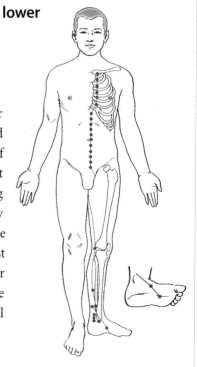

The first sign of weakening of the Kidney Meridian is pain or weakness in the back and knees. Other symptoms are dark and rough complexion, dry mouth, swollen throat, and shortness of breath. There may be loss of appetite, weakness and frequent diarrhea. In addition, the kidney is important in regulating reproductive function and urination. A simple but effective way to activate the Kidney Meridian is to hit or apply pressure to the Yong-chun points, located on the sole of the foot, with your fist or thumb. Intestine exercise is effective as well. With the lower back straight and both hands on your lower abdomen, inhale deeply and gently push your stomach out. As you exhale, pull your stomach in and imagine that it touches the spine.

9) The Pericardium Meridian must be strong for the heart to be healthy.

Pericardium Meridian

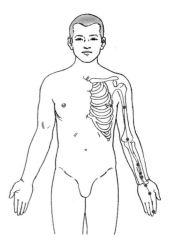

You will not find an organ called Pericardium anatomically; the pericardium is a mass of energy that wraps the heart like a scarf, thus it is often called the "heart protector." There are many symptoms common to the Heart Meridian and the Pericardium Meridian such as mental restlessness, palpitations, a flushed face, swelling or tightness in the chest and a heat sensation in the palms. For these symptoms, lightly tap the Pericardium Meridian that flows from the chest, through the middle of the inside of the arms, to the inside of the middle finger.

10) Without being an independent organ, it governs the whole body.

Triple Burner Meridian

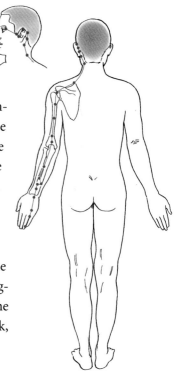

The meridian that has no shape is associated with the membrane that covers the internal organs and protects them. The upper burner, running from below the neck to below the diaphragm, the middle burner that includes the area from the diaphragm to the navel and the lower burner, running from the navel to the groin area constitute The Triple Burner. Disorder in the Triple Burner Meridian manifests as pain along the lines of ear, eye, face, jaw, neck, shoulder, arm, top of the hand and the fourth finger. A breathing method that revives the triple burner, a source of the body's energy supply, is Myung-moon breathing. Place both hands on your Dahn-jon and breathe while focusing on the Myung-moon point in the lower back, opposite the navel.

11) Stimulate the Gall Bladder Meridian to relieve migraine headache

Gall Bladder Meridian

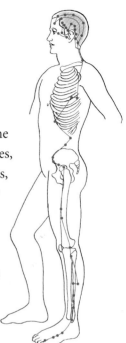

The Gall Bladder Meridian encircles a large area, from the head to the feet on both sides of the body. When you suffer from temporal headaches, migraines, or have problems in the areas of the face, ear, skin, armpits, knees, and outer legs and feet, taking good care of the Gall Bladder Meridian is very effective. Problems in the liver or the gall bladder can cause a bluish look in the whites of the eye, low energy with a feeble voice, or a high-pitched voice. For these symptoms practice Meridian exercises that stimulate the Gall Bladder Meridian flowing through the sides of the body from the outer eye to the ear, from the temple area over the top of the head to the top of the shoulder, and from the sides down to the buttocks, outer thigh, and down the leg to the fourth toes.

12) When the Liver Meridian is strong, increased stamina results

Liver Meridian

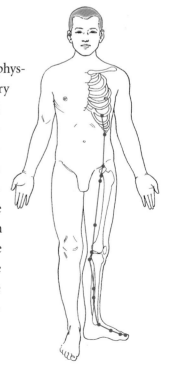

Problems with liver function can have wide-ranging effects both physically and emotionally. Symptoms may include dull complexion, dry throat, nausea and a feeling of heaviness in the chest or coastal area, anger, red painful eyes and face and a loud voice. Other symptoms include frequent diarrheas, fever and chills. Women particularly, may experience pain in the lower back and cramping in the groin area. Since the Liver Meridian connects directly to the reproductive organs in both men and women, it will be effective to use for problems related to the reproductive organs. The Liver Meridian flows from the big toe, up the foot and through the middle of the inside of each leg. With your legs stretched out, tap along the inside edge of the top of your foot, and move up to the inside of the thigh. It is also effective to tap your toe tips together while in a sitting position with your hands on your Dahn-jon.

Brain Respiration
By Ilchi Lee
Self-Training Book & CD

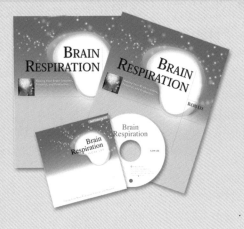

Practice Brain Respiration any time any place

Through Brain Respiration you can experience:

1. Physical coordination exercises for the body

2. Energy movement exercises for the mind

3. Awareness expanding exercises for the spirit

"In Brain Respiration, Ilchi Lee offers potent and profound methods to effect both evolutionary as well as revolutionary changes in human life and consciousness. If applied widely and seriously, the spiritual technology offered here could effect the transforming of the human condition in our time."
– Jean Houston, Ph.D Co-director of the Foundation for Mind Research

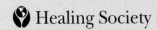

Healing Society

www.healingplaza.com e-mail:book@healingsociety.org

Healing Chakra

Light to Awaken My Soul

By Ilchi Lee

Are you happy?

This is akin to asking, "Are your Chakras healthy?"
Are you at peace?
This is also like asking, "Are your Chakras healthy?"

Chakras are the central points for the interchange
Of energy flow in our bodies.
Problems with the Chakras translate into problems
For the body, mind, and spirit.
A change in the Chakras signifies transformation
Of our body and mind.

Complete health begins and ends with the Chakras.

Healing Chakra is a simple, daily practice
to awaken your Chakra System, improve your life,
and enhance your world.

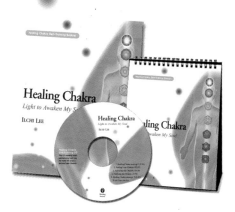

Healing Chakra Package
Includes:
Book, Self-Training CD and
Booklet

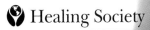
Healing Society

www.healingplaza.com e-mail:book@healingsociety.org